THE SOBER REVOLUTION

by

Sarah Turner and Lucy Rocca

Published by Accent Press Ltd – 2013

ISBN 9781783752089

This book is dedicated to every woman out there for
whom one drink is too many
and a thousand is never enough.

Acknowledgements

I could not have achieved this, my long-standing dream of writing a book, without the kind, loving and ready-at-a-second's notice support of my parents, Pam and Steve, and my sister Claire, who all stepped in to look after baby Lily whenever required.

Neither would this book have ever been finished if I had been without the encouragement and support of Sean, who believed in me from the moment we met despite the fact that on that night I was blind drunk.

Sean also provided me with one of the final pieces of my sober jigsaw, helping me realise, finally, that alcohol and I were not terribly well suited. For that moment of enlightenment I will always owe him.

To baby Lily, you can't read yet, but your arrival into my world has brought nothing but joy and happiness, and seeing your gorgeous little face each morning provides me with all the reasons I'll ever need to never drink again.

I also want to thank from the bottom of my heart, Gordon, a friend of over twenty years, who saved my life on the last night I drank alcohol.

And finally, to my ray of sunshine Isobel, for whom I wish I'd found the strength and wisdom years earlier to quit drinking (thankfully for me, she has turned out to be an angel of epic proportions and I am incredibly lucky to

call her my daughter) – thank you Isobel, for everything
(you know).

Lucy Rocca

I would like to dedicate this to my Michael – husband, best friend and rock of twenty-seven years; thank you would never cover it all. Also my son Charles, whose sense of fair-play, courage and honesty inspires me daily. I am very lucky to have lived long enough sober to show them how much they both mean to me.

Sarah Turner

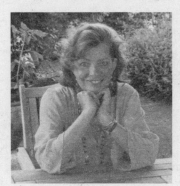
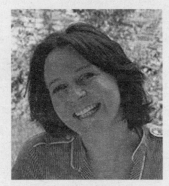

Sarah Turner   Lucy Rocca

Introduction
by Lucy Rocca

As she described to me the events of one particular night which had, like many others before it, descended into a drunken mess of staggering, screaming, self-pity and the subsequent stomach-lurching moments the morning after when, upon waking, the staccato memories had risen to the surface and she recalled some (definitely not all – the blackouts were always severe) of the terrible things she had said and done, Carol's voice was full of sad resignation. It was as though she was describing another person's life, someone whom she loved and cared for deeply but who she hadn't seen in a long time.

The summer barbeque had started out like any other; friends and family gathered for an afternoon of relaxation, good food and a few drinks in the warm sunshine. Carol, who in her own words was a greedy drunk, felt from the moment she arrived that there was only one real reason she was in attendance at this friend's convivial get-together, and it came in three colours – red, white, and rosé. Mingling amongst her friends, enjoying their company as well as the sensation of becoming slightly tipsy, Carol continued to fill her glass, gradually losing track of how much she'd had.

Unsure of when or how things suddenly switched in her head, she was told the next day how she had, after consuming many large glasses of wine, launched into tirades and abusive diatribes aimed at anyone and everyone around her. Descending into a wild and drunken rage, Carol was eventually bundled into the car with her husband and two boys and carted off back home where she could sleep it off. Upon reaching the house, however, sleep was the last thing on her mind and before long the neighbours felt justified in calling the police, concerned over the fact that Carol's two young sons were present in what appeared to be a domestic situation that was spinning rapidly out of all control.

In the mid-1990s when the barbecue incident occurred amidst numerous other regrettable drunken events, Carol was in her early thirties, mum of two sons, and caught in a marriage that was heading to an unhappy close. Her successful career placed tough demands on her which, together with the juggling of her home life and the doomed relationship which would soon end in bitter divorce, resulted in an ever-increasing affection for the wine.

As I spoke to Carol about her experiences just a few weeks before the completion of this book, it was eminently clear that I was in conversation with an articulate, confident, and sensible woman who doted on her family and valued her life, and all those who featured in it, highly. This is someone, now in her early fifties, who has recently taken up martial arts, embarked on a counselling course, has lost three stone, looks the best she has in decades and is bursting with optimism and hope for the future.

Carol's story of alcohol dependency is one which is not, sadly, uncommon. Launching into a drinking career in her twenties which took a sharp turn for the worse a decade down the line when her marriage hit the rocks and she was faced with the crippling loneliness and hardship which result from a difficult and acrimonious divorce, Carol was never a woman who could 'just have one.' As soon as the cork was popped she had her eye on what was left – would there be enough? What if it ran out? Could she justify a trip to the shop for some other imagined necessity which would enable her to slip an extra bottle into the supermarket basket – oh, so innocently, just like everyone else does?

Holding down a demanding job in which she managed hundreds of people, Carol desperately fought to maintain the façade of the 'she can have it all' 1980s mantra to friends and family. She was the life and soul, the consummate party girl, who every so often went too far and fell over the precipice into drunk and out of control.

For many who find themselves caught up in the vicious grip of an alcohol dependency, the denial is so much a part of what they are living through that it is all too easy to imagine there are no real problems caused by their drinking to excess. It is ever tempting to point at others and berate their immoral lifestyle and the effect it has on them and their families, while simultaneously wrapping ourselves in a blanket of pretence and ignoring what we are doing to our own little worlds.

As the years progressed and her drinking increased (along with the associated traumas), Carol did become aware of the impact her alcohol use may have been having on her sons.

The self-hatred and inner torment she experienced as a result of each and every awful episode fuelled by drinking led to the further erosion of Carol's inner strength and the faculties she needed so badly to sober up and dig her way out of the hole she was sinking into.

Carol did eventually put the brakes on and stopped drinking alcohol for good just over a year ago. The awful accumulation of drunken arguments, loss of self-respect, hurtful comments made which seemed to have been spoken by someone outside of her and which often she could not remember the next day, falling over, unexplained bruises, embarrassing herself in a myriad of different ways, and not being the person who she knew she was capable of being inside, eventually became too much. Carol had never descended so low as to lose her home, be disowned by her family, or sacked from her job because of her dependency on alcohol, but twenty long years of drunkenness left its scars.

For a couple of months following her bold decision to take control of her life and eradicate alcohol completely from it, Carol's relationships with her two now grown up sons improved dramatically. Both were impressed by their mum's ability to find herself amongst the wreckage of alcohol abuse, and her new upbeat mood and increased interest in their lives as opposed to being permanently side-tracked by wondering where the next glass was coming from, helped the three of them enjoy a closeness that had been missing for a while.

Last September, just a couple of months after Carol drank her last alcoholic drink, her eldest son died suddenly, aged twenty-eight. Resulting from an accidental overdose of the prescription drug Zomorph, his death came out of the blue and was horribly shocking. As I spoke to Carol about the tragedy of losing her son, I was struck by her unfaltering strength and the incredibly brave and dignified way in which she has since held the rest of the family together and remained intact for their benefit. Understanding how much it had meant to her son that she had finally managed to conquer her demons and put down the bottle, Carol explained to me how so much of her motivation for living positively and healthily now, originated in words he spoke to her just days before the end of his life; "*Mum, you not drinking is a very good thing.*"

Carol is well aware that should she resume the destructive

relationship she once had with alcohol she would not be the person she is today; with her hope and courage, together with all the ample time and energy she is now able to spend on those around her, Carol's *raison d'être* is to claw back the life she lost to drinking for so many years and to give back whatever she can. Knowing that her son spent precious time with her in the final months of his life during which she was free from the grip of alcohol and all of its soul-destroying effects, gives Carol some comfort in the tragic aftermath of his death.

It has become blindingly clear to her that upon escaping the alcohol trap, the world opens up. Ruminating over the pointlessness of consuming all that wine could be enough to make a lesser person sink, but Carol has found the strength to fight, carving out a new and meaningful existence of which her son would be proud. There are no longing glances at a guest's glass of wine across the dining table, or feelings of resentment towards her hugely supportive partner for his desire to have a couple of glasses before dinner; Carol has thrown herself headlong into the wonderful world of sobriety and is relishing all the positivity that it has introduced into her life.

Fully aware of the fact that sobriety is an all or nothing prize, of the impossibility of reaping the many rewards that are derived from an alcohol-free life without committing to it one hundred per cent, Carol is in this for the long haul.

Looking back over her lifetime, she is now able to extract the good and employ it as the foundations for even better, while simultaneously accepting she will never change what's been and gone. The wonderfully positive characteristics that emanate from Carol, despite all she has faced in the last twelve months, are what led me to asking her if I could share her story for the purpose of this introduction. In my opinion, she embodies all that it is to love life, in control.

Carol is one of many women who unwittingly slip into the realms of alcohol dependency, so busy with attempting to keep the many plates of their lives spinning that they fail to notice how the pleasant glass of wine after the kids have been put to bed slowly transforms into a much-needed crutch, longingly lusted after throughout each and every hectic day. People who wind up with a 'drinking problem' are, for the most part, a long way off the archetypal drunk sleeping on a park bench with an oversized bottle of cheap cider to hand. Those who struggle with an alcohol dependency are everyday people who once 'enjoyed a drink' but for whom gradually the alluring qualities of booze are replaced by something much more sinister.

Pigeon-holing very heavy drinkers as 'alcoholics' is an easy way to deflect the accusatory finger away from one's own destructive relationship with booze – *'I never drink before tea-time'* and *'I never touch spirits'* being commonly used reassurances which prevent people from facing up to the fact that they are, in actual fact, alcohol-dependent.

Because I never considered myself to be 'an alcoholic' I failed to pay much attention to how dangerously unhealthy my wine habit had become. My daughter was never under threat of being taken into care, I had a nice place to live and was never in a position where I couldn't pay the mortgage, and I still looked reasonably OK, as the really obvious visible signposting of physical damage caused by excessive alcohol consumption becomes far more apparent further down the line. I stopped drinking alcohol aged thirty-five, and had only recently begun to notice during the previous couple of years the more prominent and difficult-to-hide facial indicators of being hung-over; the ruddy complexion, sallow skin, sunken eyes and overly red lips becoming regular features of my appearance as my drinking reached epic proportions.

At my worst I was consuming around one hundred and fifty units per week, which equates to one or two bottles of wine a night with a few extra drinks thrown in at the weekend. Even then, I did not feel constantly alarmed at the amount I was drinking – rather I was occasionally beset (usually upon waking in the middle of the night) by a terribly morbid fear that I was killing myself slowly, and that any day I would find a lump somewhere on my person, the indicator of a lifestyle-induced cancer. But for the most part I threw caution to the wind and continued apace with socialising, boozing, and living in denial.

I consumed my last drink in April 2011, and since then have rediscovered the person I am. It is only with complete sobriety that I have come to realise just how much of the real me I sacrificed in exchange for alcohol.

I grew up wanting to be a writer. I loved reading and ploughed my way through *Watership Down* and *Jane Eyre* before I reached my teens. Scattered amongst the belongings in my bedroom were scores of notebooks filled with scribbles and doodles, little ideas for stories that popped into my head constantly. It never occurred to me that I wouldn't one day write a book or become a journalist when I grew up.

And then I discovered drinking. Alcohol had many negative effects on my life during the twenty years in which I consumed it excessively, but one thing it robbed me of which I am especially grateful to have rediscovered as a result of becoming alcohol-free, is my creativity. It is only with sober hindsight that I can truly appreciate just how barren my life had become as a result of my on-going drunkenness, where the only interest I had outside of my family and job was drinking.

Living in the UK and growing up amongst a culture which positively celebrates alcohol, spending my weekends inebriated was a completely expected part of life, and I never imagined for a moment that I would not jump on board the drunken merry-go-round along with everyone else. My friends all drank regularly, boyfriends were always heavy drinkers and so I found myself easily drawn into a habit of emotional and mental alcohol dependence which was, unfortunately, to last for two decades.

At the time of writing I have not touched alcohol for twenty-six months and I have never been happier, more positive or so full of self-confidence, more productive, a better and more capable mother or in such good physical shape. In a relatively short space of time my life has completely turned around and I owe it to the simple act of choosing to not drink alcohol.

Shortly after Soberistas.com was launched in November 2012, I was contacted by an addiction counsellor and cognitive behavioural therapist called Sarah Turner. After successfully turning her own life around after years of abusing alcohol, Sarah retrained and became a qualified practitioner, enabling her to establish the Harrogate Sanctuary in 2006 which offers women a guiding light out of the gloom of alcohol addiction. Sarah read about Soberistas in a newspaper and recognised immediately that we both had a keen desire to offer help and support to the same demographic; grown-up women who had hit the bottle hard in their efforts to cope with life's struggles.

A few months after our initial meeting Sarah and I agreed upon the idea of putting a book together that would offer practical help for beating an alcohol dependency, based on our own personal experiences. Our collaboration would be much more than a standard self-help book, however, in that it would also include real life case studies of women (and one of a married couple) who have battled their demons and emerged out of the other side shining. The sense of optimism and inspiration that can be derived from reading about people who once felt deeply unhappy and desperate as a consequence of alcohol but who, through a variety of different methods eventually resolved their difficulties, can be vast and incredibly motivating.

Sarah and I both perceive our troubled drinking histories as akin to doomed love affairs – in our efforts to acquire self-confidence and be loved and comforted, we increasingly turned to the bottle hoping the hollowness in our lives could somehow be filled by the liquid inside. Drinking and getting drunk perpetually for years, the drawn out battles we were engaged in with alcohol were not dissimilar to some of the unsatisfactory love affairs with men that marked our late teens and early twenties. As the relationship progressed, the booze took more and more and we lost all sense of our identities, emotional strength, and the ability to walk away. Alcohol gradually transformed the both of us from strong and feisty women who knew exactly what we wanted from life, to a pair of weak-willed, powerless nobodies whose only care in the world was where the next drink was coming from.

For me, coming of age during the 'ladette' years when it was suddenly de rigueur to neck pints on a night out in an effort to keep up with the lads, meant that my lack of awareness in recognising when I'd had enough to drink, and my desire to consume alcohol to the point of collapse, both went largely unnoticed. I simply blended in with a social group of hedonistic boozers who thought absolutely nothing of drinking for twelve hours straight.

It was many years later before I came to notice that the people around me no longer appeared to spend their entire weekends getting sloshed, and for most, being seen to be blatantly drunk was an embarrassment that they would attempt to avoid at all costs. Despite the awareness that I grew to have of people generally frowning on those who fall out of taxis blind drunk, engage in loud nonsensical arguments in the street or throw up loudly in a pub toilet, slumped on the floor and hanging onto the porcelain for dear life, I still maintained my reputation as something of 'a liability' on a night out.

Try as I might to instil some rules with regards to the amount or type of drink that I consumed, I pretty much always ended up absolutely plastered, my memory blacked out, and nothing but self-hatred and regrets the morning after. Despite years of trying, I never managed to moderate my alcohol consumption, and eventually arrived at the conclusion that for me, it was all or nothing. I chose nothing, which in the event has turned out to be my all.

I succeeded, as did Sarah, at conquering my alcohol addiction because I ultimately accepted the truth that if the agony of destructive drinking can ever come to an end, it has to be replaced by a solid commitment to *not drinking*. Obvious as that may sound, many people reach the decision that their relationship with alcohol is unhealthy and must be addressed, that they no longer wish to suffer all the associated awfulness of regular binge drinking, while simultaneously hoping against hope that somehow they will be able to manage their problem through control and moderation.

The vast number of people who have wiped out years of their lives through the misguided belief that alcohol is serving a purpose (stress reliever, relaxant, mood enhancer) when in actuality it is responsible for robbing them of their self-confidence, self-esteem, happiness and ability to view the world unhampered by blinkers, is staggering. For so many, the fact that they have yet to characterise themselves as 'an alcoholic' because they have not lost their worldly possessions or resorted to sleeping on a park bench means they allow themselves to spin out the delusion a little while longer – that they are in control of alcohol and not the other way around.

Adopting a lifestyle of sobriety restores the mind and body to what they once were, and allows us to fill the shoes of the person we were born to be. Making the choice to stop drinking alcohol means empowering one's self; taking charge of one's own life and ensuring a much greater degree of emotional stability, which will impact positively on those closest to us. Ditching the demon drink means walking away from the endless cycle of negativity and bashing of self – the mornings filled with recriminations and self-hatred, when the only option appears to be hiding under the duvet and wishing the world would disappear, will vanish without a trace, never to be seen again.

In writing this book we have no desire to appear evangelical, and recognise that there are many people in this world who enjoy a drink and are able to have fun with it. However, our intention is to show that life is not the boring and dull existence so often portrayed by society when depicting those who choose to not drink alcohol. Just as drunks are stigmatized, often so are non-drinkers; they are frequently considered odd, perhaps once weak-minded or unable to let their hair down, rather than people who are in control and able to fulfil their true potential.

Throughout the following chapters you will read the remarkable stories of women who eventually arrived at the conclusion that a life minus alcohol had to be better than the continuation of the booze-inflicted misery in which they had been drowning for so long. Despite, for all, an initial terror at the prospect of a life spent separated from their one true love, alcohol, all nine of the case studies ultimately arrived at the conclusion that they only really embarked upon the act of living once the wine had been kicked out of their lives for good. Seven of the women whose stories are featured in this book are previous clients of Sarah who kindly, and very bravely, agreed to Sarah writing up her case notes on each of them, in order to create a powerful collection of real life recovery tales.

During the 1990s, feminism for me was best illustrated by the fact that women could happily prop up the bar next to any number of men and smoke and drink pints with them all evening. Now in my late thirties, I consider alcohol to be the key factor in the transformation of my personality from strong and full of gumption in my teens, to depressed, anxiety-ridden, and severely lacking in self-confidence and self-belief by my early thirties – a fine example of anti-feminism.

The love/hate relationship that so many people endure with alcohol is surely nothing but the antithesis to nurturing a happy existence in which we fulfil our potential and maximise the opportunities which surround us from the moment we are born. Becoming dependent on alcohol leads to a dead end; a horribly predictable negative cycle where nothing ever improves and the same mistakes are made over and over again.

In writing this book, Sarah and I set out to describe a mindset which we believe is the key to successfully walking away from a destructive relationship with alcohol. By fully acknowledging the fact that alcohol adds nothing to your life and is actually responsible for preventing you from reaching self-fulfilment, it *is* possible to break the long-standing drinking patterns that become so innocuously entrenched in our lives.

If one embarks on alcohol-free living with the deep-seated belief that they've given up something of worth then they are heading for a resounding fall from the wagon. To conquer alcohol-dependency, it is crucial never to consider one's self to be '*on the wagon*' in the first place; this expression is loaded with connotations of temporariness, a short-term quiescence from normal life. In order to walk away from booze for good, it is essential that upon reaching this incredibly positive and empowering decision, you recognise that it is a step which will lead you to great things, the beginning of an exciting adventure and a whole new way of life.

What you are NOT doing is giving up a treat and choosing to live your life like a hermit who can have no fun; you are resurrecting the old you from the wasteland of drink-fuelled misery and discovering what the world is really about, minus the booze blinkers that have kept you submerged for so long.

This book came about as a result of both Sarah's and my perception of our erstwhile relationships with alcohol being similar in many ways to doomed love affairs, and because we believe that becoming alcohol-free is a lifestyle choice that demands commitment right from the start. There will be bad days and good days (over time the good most definitely outweigh the bad), rocky patches and feelings of doubt, but ultimately, empowering yourself by ditching alcohol can only come about if you stick with your decision.

In this way we believe that committing to sobriety resembles, in many ways, the personal investment many people put into a long-term relationship.

Imagine finding a partner who makes you feel wonderful

every day – who boosts your self-esteem, makes you feel confident and self-assured, is financially stable, fires up your passion for life, encourages your productivity, supports your endeavours to be a great parent, pampers you, encourages you to take good care of yourself by eating the right foods and exercising, and guides you along a path of self-discovery.

This person would nurture your character, never trying to sway you to be someone you aren't. He would make you see that you are uniquely perfect, someone to be cherished and celebrated. He would acknowledge your flaws but accept and love them as a part of you, as imperfections of a perfect one-off – you.

If you could drop yourself into a world in which this person not only exists but is also ready and waiting for you to be by his side for ever, would you contemplate making a commitment to him? If all of the above was guaranteed to be yours for as long as you were prepared to stay true to our imaginary Mr Wonderful, would you make the leap of faith and say yes?

In this book you will read about a lifestyle choice that is simple to make, relatively easy to stick to and guaranteed to provide you with the tools required for a real and positive state of being. It's a choice that you may have dabbled with the idea of for years, never quite knowing whether to make the final leap, or perhaps it's something that you have only recently been considering. Either way, if you continue to read on, you will find out that the choice of sobriety is the lifestyle equivalent of our imaginary Mr Wonderful, and it is yours for the taking.

All you have to do is say YES.

We know this book can help you make the decision to quit

drinking. It will help you start on a very liberating journey. Please take a moment to reflect on how you are feeling about your relationship with alcohol.

- How are you feeling right now?

- Are you worried about how much you drink?

- Have you been suffering health effects from your drinking?

- Has your relationship with family and friends been impacted by your drink?

- Is it causing you problems at work?

- Would it help your finances if you stopped spending money on alcohol?

- Are you fed up with losing control?

The Sober Revolution

Part One,
by Lucy Rocca

CHAPTER ONE –
Flirting With the Notion of Sobriety

For many people, alcohol has the same draw as a particularly charming yet dangerous lover; its surface attraction beguiling a hidden hotbed of deceit, unpredictability and destruction. For all those wonderful nights spent sharing a bottle of wine with friends or a partner, nibbling on tasty finger foods by candlelight and talking amiably until the cows come home, there are a plethora of arguments, ill-advised 'romantic' trysts, wine-induced carb-fests resulting in difficult-to-shift spare tyres, mornings of recriminations and self-hatred, outrageous flirtations with people not to be flirted with, embarrassing stumbles outside crowded bars and slurred, drunken behaviour in front of the kids which demands an explanation in the morning through the fog of a hangover.

And for all of the above less than charming repercussions of excessive alcohol consumption, a little thing called denial will persistently try to work its magic, persuading you to focus on the positives and ignore the ever-increasing list of negatives in order to keep you pouring.

I began drinking in my early teens. Growing up in a middle-class family with teachers for parents, a large house in the suburbs, and the requisite black Labrador, I hailed from a secure and totally functional background. I have no particular excuses for embarking upon an exceptionally destructive relationship with wine (and beer and spirits when the wine ran dry) other than it's what teenagers did in suburban Sheffield in the late 1980s.

We loitered around the school grounds on warm summer evenings, smoking Marlboros, listening to The Smiths and drinking expensive bottles of Claret or Pinot Noir stolen from various friends' affluent parents' wine cellars. As the years passed by my friends changed in person but not in type and I continued to socialise with those who 'liked a drink.' It was therefore never forefront in my mind that I drank too much or that I (heaven forbid!) might have a dependency on booze.

In the halcyon years of my late teens and twenties, long before the idea of my own mortality had raised its gloomy head and I lived beneath a sun that apparently would never set, risks to personal health posed by fun and outrageous nights spent drinking purely to get drunk, puffing away on cigarettes with as much concern as if they were the confectionary version bought for a penny as a child, it was easy to float along, quietly developing an emotional dependency on alcohol without realising it.

Beneath my outward recklessness, however, I did read and latch onto fixedly the news stories which began to emerge in the early 1990s regarding red wine and how it allegedly had health benefits. Following the US news programme 60 Minutes airing a story entitled 'French Paradox' which highlighted the low incidence rate of heart disease amongst the French despite their love of high fat and dairy foods, pointing to their equal love of vin rouge as an explanation for this, the US saw sales of red wine jump by 44% over previous years. The story quickly found its way across the Atlantic, helping to reassure the boozy

17

Britons that they too were being good to themselves by drinking all that alcohol.

The Mediterranean diet, all those gloriously healthy Tuscans drinking their Chianti and scoffing beans, artichokes, and olives under a baking Italian sun – somewhere in my befuddled mind I adopted the belief that I too was buying into such a life each time I dropped a nice bottle of red into my shopping trolley along with some antipasti and a selection of artisan breads.

But the fact that I was cherry-picking the positive news stories regarding drinking habits and choosing to ignore the less reassuring ones would suggest that as far back as fifteen years prior to my stopping drinking alcohol altogether, I had begun to worry about my wine habit just a little.

So what might cause you to have concerns over the amount of alcohol you are consuming? You, your friends, and partner all drink at every social event you attend, occasionally becoming inebriated, rowdy, and a little irresponsible. The hangovers have always been a constant presence since you began drinking and are therefore part and parcel of this ubiquitous and very accepted form of substance abuse that you regularly partake in, but recently they have become somewhat debilitating resulting in you spending half the weekend in bed. The panic attacks and state of paranoia that you suffer following particularly heavy drinking episodes may have become more intense and are occurring with an increased frequency, and perhaps you have begun to regularly experience memory blackouts.

Despite all of the negative consequences that occur as a direct result of the alcohol that you drink, you have most likely become something of a con artist to yourself, developing a brilliantly honed technique of denial and preferred ignorance over the years which affords you room to drink undeterred by worry. That is, until the morning after when you are plagued with the fear, depression, and sinking regrets over what you did the night before.

It is a common phenomenon that finds most regular binge drinkers clutching their head in woe on a Saturday or Sunday morning, despairing of their actions from the previous night's activities and swearing to themselves and anyone else who will listen that they will never touch the stuff again – only to repeat their actions the following weekend.

As a regular binge-drinker you will more than likely have toyed with the idea of giving up alcohol time and time again. It's an easy little plaything, one that doesn't demand any real commitment or thinking time but a fleeting thought of 'Maybe I'll stop drinking for a while.'

Imagine that alcohol is a particularly unsuitable lover who you know is no good for you. Although you recognise him as an ill match, he is charming and persuasive and despite the fact that your evenings often end in rows you can't help getting in touch with him again as soon as things blow over, your faithful return as predictable as a boomerang's. Over and over again the same pattern plays out; you meet, you have fun, you fight, you part company, you make up, you have earth-shattering sex, you cuddle, you fight, and around and around you go.

I had a relationship like this soon after my divorce in my late twenties. The man in question was as handsome as they come, we had a lot of fun, and we were very physically attracted to each other. But there the positive connections ended leaving little else to glue us together as a couple. In my head I knew I should break up with him, but the lure of him and the law of attraction kept on pulling me back for approximately a year.

19

Eventually I saw sense and we split up for good, but saying goodbye to him was not dissimilar to ending other addictions I have battled and eventually conquered. I had to adjust to filling my time with other things; I had to find alternative sources of comfort whenever I craved a cuddle or a boost to my flailing ego.

Many people are addicted to the drama and topsy-turvy chaos that heavy alcohol consumption brings with it – even if they don't know it. Regularly getting drunk usually means engaging in one or more of the following; messing up relationships, breaking promises, being reckless, coping with huge shame and regret, flirting with strangers, having affairs, making impetuous decisions, and acting upon whimsical, romantic notions that seem like a great idea after too many glasses of Pinot Grigio. Frequently getting sloshed is not dissimilar to being involved with a wayward and thoroughly unsuitable partner – you want him and then he lets you down, over and over again.

What starts off as an exciting union of passion and hotbed of thrills slowly dwindles into a boring, repetitive cycle of crazed pleasure-seeking, dampened swiftly by a blanket of regret.

Partners who turn out to be unsuitable do not usually reveal themselves as such in the first instance. When you initially began to drink alcohol you probably enjoyed the buzz it gave you, the sense of abandonment and possibly the feelings of sexual confidence that led you to being rather more flirtatious than usual, less shy around someone you fancied. You may have continued to experience such pleasant reactions every time you drank alcohol for quite some time, years perhaps.

Similarly, a person who eventually reveals his self to be completely not your cup of tea is usually perceived as the total opposite in the early weeks and sometimes months of the relationship. Often it is the case that we do not even recognise when someone is having a destructive and negative effect on our lives, caught up as we are in the frenetic and emotional rush of a fresh new romance. And when the day finally dawns when we do come to realise that this person who we thought was so perfect for us once upon a time is actually totally unsuitable, it can prove difficult to give them the boot and move onto someone more reliable and steady, intertwined as we are by then in a web of emotional dependencies.

Many people enjoy the excitement of a bad lover; the ups and downs, the terrible fights followed by the passionate making up are perceived as utterly worth it when we are madly in love. If you have an emotional dependency on alcohol then the thought of giving up all that recklessness, the sense of throwing caution to the wind as the first glass slips down after a long, gruelling day, the sophisticated way you feel when you sip champagne from a cut crystal flute dressed in a pretty dress and heels – relinquishing all of that for a more steady and predictable life, sober, can be a hard concept to grasp.

When we pour that first drink of the evening we are saying to those around us, "This is my time now; I'm here, but this is Mummy's wine o'clock, Mummy's special time and you need to respect that." The wine is a prop that demarcates the end of the hustle and bustle of the day and the beginning of the grown-up, relaxed affair that is evening. That first glass is the longed-for rendezvous with Mr Unsuitable, after a day spent bogged down with the humdrum of domesticity and/or work.

The regret-laden hangover which presents itself the morning after a heavy night of binge-drinking is often severe enough to warrant a short-lived dalliance with the idea of becoming teetotal, just as an evening spent arguing with your dangerous bad boy lover may cause you to debate the idea of finishing with him once and for all and finding a nice dependable type instead – you find yourself craving some stability and reliability in your life. It's a pleasant thought that makes you feel back in control of your life, and your imagination runs wild for a while with the idea of settling down and being happy and content.

I have lost count of the number of times I considered giving up alcohol, of saying goodbye to my own Mr Wrong. There was the morning after the night when I was so drunk I fell into the (empty) bath while brushing my teeth, banging my head and waking a very unsympathetic ex-partner from his slumber with the crash; another morning when I awoke to the awful stench of hours-old vomit, opening my eyes to see the puke-stained carpet next to my side of the bed, scrubbed but ruined for ever by the bin lid sized circle of orange-coloured sick I had expelled a few hours earlier while asleep; the day after a huge row with an ex had prompted a passer-by to conclude that I was the subject of domestic violence (I wasn't) and to launch himself on my ex in some misguided effort to protect me – the ex-boyfriend wound up being arrested and thrown into cells for the night, the police remaining unconvinced of his innocence despite my drunken protestations of the reverse.

After these and countless other alcohol-fuelled disastrous events I would wake up with an almighty hangover, the pounding in my head soon fading into insignificance as the overwhelming sense of dread and fear rose from the pit of my stomach and began to spread its icy chill throughout every inch of my being. Consumed by self-hatred and remorse I would promise myself 'never again,' make a cup of tea, curl up in front of the TV and wait for the awfulness to subside.

A couple of days later I would be making my next wine purchase and reassuring myself that this time it would be different.

The reasons behind this yo-yoing between heavy binge-drinking and sobriety, of drifting back and forth between a dependable Mr Darcy and the archetypal bad boy Daniel Cleaver (Bridget Jones' Diary) are often down to drama; put very simply, some people like the excitement of it all. The short-lived intention to 'behave ourselves' and quit alcohol never lasts longer than a few days because the steady pace of living alcohol-free seems boring in comparison, and we revert back to our old ways in an effort to reignite the flame of excitement that we feel has been put out.

However, there comes a point in many people's lives when the rollercoaster thrills we welcomed as they hit us thick and fast in our younger years suddenly become tiring, leaving us weary in their wake. The repercussions of a drunken night out are no longer so easy to brush off; the after-effects of our flirtatious, maybe unfaithful behaviour as a result of drinking too much are far-reaching and destructive – lives are being affected and not just our own. Our health becomes more of a concern as we mature and come to terms with the idea of our own mortality and we feel as though something must change; we begin to consider other options. We flirt a little more seriously with the idea of getting our alcohol consumption under control.

A common first step is the intention of instilling boundaries in order to limit the amount we drink, thus putting some damage limitation measures into place. With a wayward boyfriend these limitations might be that we will only see him at the weekend, we will make an effort to cool off emotionally to avoid further dependency, or perhaps we might consider giving him an ultimatum – behave yourself or we're finished.

In replacing the disrespectful lover with alcohol, those same boundaries are equally applicable. Some of my own rules that I attempted to enforce as a regular drinker included no wine when out drinking with friends (large pub measures would usually result in more extreme and rapid drunkenness than if I stuck to beer), no drinking mid-week (except Wednesdays when my daughter went to stay the night at her dad's) and no more than a bottle of wine in one sitting. I never stuck to any of them, and so the madness would continue.

I would also occasionally embark on a 'detox' in the misguided belief that a few weeks off the sauce would aid my poor liver's recovery; the idea that stopping drinking for a month or two can be of help to a damaged liver is nonsense – the only way to avoid alcohol-related liver damage is either to drink very moderately (i.e. sticking to government guidelines) or abstaining completely.

The alcoholic take on 'let's have some thinking space' is not an entire waste of effort or time, however. Living without alcohol for the rest of your life can seem to many people a daunting prospect. Despite the fact that you have a growing awareness of the fact that you and alcohol are a bad match and are destined for a perpetual rocky road, choosing to remain sober permanently can be perceived as a move into scary and virgin territory, and something that you simply cannot contemplate doing for the rest of your life.

A few weeks or maybe months spent without alcohol can bring to the fore all the positives of choosing sobriety as a way of life. Better sleep, improved skin, weight loss, eradication of mood swings, heightened productivity, being a more patient and energetic parent, and feeling calmer and better able to cope in stressful situations are all positive side-effects of not drinking. Perhaps allowing yourself time for a sabbatical from your boozy lifestyle is a good starting point if you know that you need to regain control of your life with regards to alcohol but aren't quite ready to take the big step to a lifetime commitment yet.

If you embark on this short-term approach be sure to keep a record of how living without alcohol makes you feel, including both pros and cons; having a tangible list in black and white to return to whenever you need a reminder can help you put things into perspective, as well as deciding on how to proceed with your relationship with drinking. In the build-up to your temporary break, keep a drinks diary too – people regularly underestimate how much alcohol they are consuming, but by keeping a record of this you are arming yourself with the facts you need when making future decisions.

In regarding alcohol as a particularly undesirable partner we can draw comparisons which should highlight why you would be better off living without it, although you would more than likely have seen these from a mile off if we were talking about an unsuitable human partner.

In a relationship, how long would you be prepared to stand for the following; a lover who repeatedly puts you down and in doing so gradually erodes your self-confidence, one who encourages you to lose interest in any worthwhile activities that you may once have had, who tries to come between you and your kids with the effect that your parenting skills are significantly lessened, someone who encourages you to eat badly and do little exercise with the end result being weight gain and lack of fitness, a partner who keeps you awake at night jibing you with negative thoughts and preventing you from obtaining your optimum eight hours of sleep leaving you irritable and unable to concentrate at work the following day? How would you react if a partner did all of these things to you and in return for this inventory of misery you received only the following positive effects from his company?

The very occasional night of fun, untainted by arguments, jealousy, or any other negativity, and an hour or two of excited anticipation leading up to each rendezvous?

It is likely that you would dump him without a second thought.

In contemplating breaking up with a partner, particularly one who has damaged our self-esteem, leaving us feeling unconfident and emotionally bruised, we often experience self-doubt and anxieties with regards to the unknown territory of our single futures. Once the deed has been done, however, we rarely continue to suffer such crippling emotional uncertainties and after a couple of weeks pick ourselves up and get back in the race – to quote Frank Sinatra.

After ridding ourselves of an unsatisfactory relationship that has pulled us down for a while and caused much unhappiness, it can be a blessed relief to finally give the son of a b**ch the heave-ho for good.

In our new found singledom, it is not unusual to rediscover the activities we so enjoyed prior to meeting Mr Wrong, meet up once more with neglected friends, buy some new clothes, and enjoy an overall feeling of joie de vivre; and all this when prior to ending the relationship we were terrified of feeling alone and depressed for the rest of our lives!

So, you have endured a rough time with alcohol and you now deem your long-standing emotional crutch to be thoroughly unsuitable and unworthy of your attentions – it's time to move on. Even though life without the prop of alcohol can present itself as a metaphorical leap off a cliff into a massive dark hole, it is important to remind yourself at this point of a very definite truth – things can only get better once you have kicked Mr Unsuitable into touch!

Soberistas is where you can meet people who are trying to resolve their problematic drinking patterns, and people who have successfully kicked the booze.

Talk, write, offload, share —join Soberistas and let's change together, today.

CHAPTER TWO

Your Choice to Make a Positive Commitment

For years you have tussled with the thought that you and alcohol do not form a good match – there have been too many mornings of regret, too many broken promises that you would end the relationship for good, and way too much misery which has come about as a direct result of this destructive union. My own realisation of how things between me and alcohol were heading down a sad one-way road to a bleak future came about over the space of a couple of years prior to me eventually calling time on my alcohol dependency for ever.

At first it was the odd thought pertaining to sobriety but gradually over the months the signs grew stronger and eventually I faced the truth square in the face and with no more excuses; if I didn't stop drinking alcohol I would never be happy.

Making the decision to move on with my life was brought to a head following a particularly excessive night of binge-drinking which I undertook alone in my old apartment. My daughter was staying at her dad's for the night, my new boyfriend was out with friends and I made the choice to buy three bottles of wine. I drank them all plus a bottle of cider that had been lurking in my fridge for a few weeks (I hate cider – someone else had bought it and very kindly left it for me one night!), took the dog up the drive so that she could have a wee and I could have a cigarette, and there I collapsed and began throwing up relentlessly while unconscious on the pavement at 10 o'clock at night.

Thankfully for me a friend was serendipitously driving past on his motorbike and happened to see both me and the poor little dog standing by my side looking confused. He called an ambulance and the next thing I was aware of was waking up under the bright lights of a hospital A&E ward covered in congealed sick. Lovely. I guess this was the alcohol equivalent of finally acknowledging the unsuitability of a particularly troublesome partner after they lose their temper and proceed to beat you up mercilessly – it was a case of 'Oh, I get it – if I hang around with you any longer you will kill me.' And there ended my relationship with alcohol after twenty long years.

Because there was no other way, I jumped straight into a dalliance with sobriety but for a long time there was a big part of me who wasn't keen on the idea at all. I did not make a completely happy commitment to this new way of life, rather I felt as though my hand had been forced out of a desire to not die. On occasion, I missed my old beau dreadfully and harboured the odd thought of nipping up to the shop to buy in a bottle of my poison. There were times when I found it difficult to contemplate that I would spend the rest of my days miserably separated from my one true love.

That being said, I also felt a large element of relief and a sense of freedom in the first few weeks of sobriety. The mornings devoid of crippling hangovers and fear over something I may have said/texted/done the night before while drunk were fresh and welcomed after years of carrying a heavy burden on my shoulders of anxiety and dread.

For me the biggest difficulty in stopping drinking was not the actual physical act of no longer imbibing alcohol, but learning to appreciate and love a life without it in order to prevent any desire to start knocking the wine back again. I had (ab)used alcohol for over two decades to numb every emotion from happiness to sadness. I had drunk at each and every celebration and social event that I had ever attended, ensuring that I had no idea how to converse confidently without this social lubricant that I had unwittingly relied on so heavily for such a long time.

Ending my destructive partnership with alcohol left me feeling utterly lost and terrified of what lay before me. It was as if I had finally unlocked my prison cell door only to reveal complete blackness, a vacuum devoid of anything which may act as a hint of what the future holds. The emotional blindness I experienced was crippling – I had no clue which way to turn for fear that I may fall off the edge into an abyss. I was filled with a huge sense of shame and a morbid self-hatred owing to my last fling with alcohol and because of the multitude of regretful incidents that I had lived through over the years as a result of being drunk. For days I remained indoors whenever possible, too scared to go out in case I saw someone I knew and would then have to speak to.

With my confidence at an all-time low I muddled along, keeping my head down and my eye on the prize – a life that did not involve any more drunken mayhem and subsequently, a better life for my daughter. I was correct to remind myself of the idiom 'This too will pass,' because eventually it did. Finally, after many weeks of hiding from both myself and my feelings, I saw the first weak rays of sunlight lighting up the dark space before me. I began to notice the very faintest of paths and my feet immediately found their way to following it.

If you are now in the transitional period between your acceptance of the fact that you and alcohol are not a match made in heaven and that you wish very strongly to never drink again, and establishing a happy union with sobriety, you will more than likely be feeling lost and uncertain of how to proceed. I have included an article below from Soberistas.com which you should read now to remind yourself of why you should stick with your plan to quit drinking and engage with the idea of sobriety.

"I'm 37 years old and struggled with depression, anxiety and the odd panic attack for twenty years of my life, prior to April 2011. My nerves frequently got the better of me, and my obvious lack of confidence in work and social situations held me back and prevented me from fulfilling my potential for many years. If you had asked me to describe my personality a couple of years ago, I would have responded with a jumbled, insecure answer; unsure of who I really was, full of pretence as to the person I wanted to be, knowing that inside I didn't particularly like myself but not fully realising how to change. All of that stopped when I quit drinking alcohol two years ago.

If you have a sneaky suspicion that alcohol is controlling you a little more than you feel comfortable with then read on – this may be the first step you have subconsciously wanted to take for a long time.

If you binge drink and subsequently get drunk a lot you will, whoever you are, occasionally make an idiot of yourself. You will say stupid things, have unnecessary arguments, fall over, lose your phone or handbag, text someone who you really shouldn't, make sexual advances towards a person who is, how shall I put this ..? Not quite at your usual standard. You may even put your safety at risk, walking home late at night alone, slightly wobbly, looking like an easy target for an attacker, or drink so much that you are sick after you have fallen asleep. Every time that you wake up the morning after a session where one or several of the above have occurred, your self-esteem will take a bit of a battering. Multiply those beatings by each weekend/night/day that you binge drink and you will appreciate that your self-respect and self-esteem are severely and negatively affected by alcohol.

Alcohol depresses the central nervous system. Physiologically, that anxiety and nervy disposition that you, as a regular binge drinker, have probably noticed is increasing with age, is down to booze. When I drank, I had frequent panic attacks, the last one being so severe that I thought I was dying. I had to walk out of the packed cinema in which I was trying to watch The King's Speech because I was fighting to breathe. It was hours later until I regained my normal composure, and days until I fully recovered from the fright and trauma that I suffered as a result of thinking that I was on my way to meeting my maker. The reason behind this anxiety attack was that I had drunk too much beer the night before.

For years I pin-balled between unsuitable relationships; one boyfriend would have the physical attributes I was looking for, but not the mental compatibility. I would dump the first one and jump straight in to another union with someone who had the brains and emotional energy I was after, but who, after time, I had no physical connection with whatsoever. I couldn't be alone. My depression and low self-esteem meant that I constantly needed the reassurance of being in a relationship just to feel wanted and loved. I was incapable of loving myself. Alcohol kept me from being in a happy and balanced relationship with a person who loves me as much as I love them.

Drinking put me in a perpetual state of either a) being drunk or b) being hungover. Neither of these conditions is conducive to a productive, fulfilling life. My career, financial wellbeing, and physical fitness were all below par (by a long way) when I drank. I am not a lazy person but I never achieved much during the years in which I got drunk. Since giving up drinking, my achievements just keep on growing each week – in turn this boosts my self-esteem and belief in what I am capable of. And so I keep on achieving and aiming higher.

Without drink in my life, my anxiety and narcissistic tendencies have vanished, and guess what? I like myself! And the natural conclusion to that, of course, is that other people like me more too. I have finally found a man who I think is perfect (for me, at least), and we have a wonderful family life which I value above anything else. I am running regularly and am the fittest I have ever been. My relationship with my eldest daughter (at that tricky teenage stage) is great, and we are very close. I have bags of energy (essential for looking after my one-year-old properly), and squeeze masses into each and every day. I never stay in bed, idling away those precious hours that could be spent on accomplishing something worthwhile. My skin and general appearance have improved, my eyes are bright and I don't have to fight to keep a beer belly at bay. I am happy, the happiest I have ever been in my life, and this is down to one simple fact – I gave up booze.

This account of all the positives to be gained in ditching alcohol are very real and not to be sniffed at in favour of your misguided belief that next time you meet up with Mr Vino things will be different; they won't. Moderation works only for people who do not have an emotional or physical dependency on alcohol, and no one else. And if you did not have an emotional or physical dependency on booze, then it is unlikely you would be reading this book.

If you are anything like me then in your younger years (or maybe more recently) you will have been involved with, and then departed company from, a lover who was not best suited to you. Some partners, particularly those Daniel Cleaver types, can be especially difficult to stay away from once the decision to make the break has been made.

I recall one such ex-boyfriend of mine who, following a lengthy and loud argument at my parents' house where I was still living at the time (I was sixteen), I informed that if he walked out the door I would never see or speak to him again. Obviously, he walked out of the door. In a state of heart-broken desperation and unable to find a pair of shoes in sufficient time to catch him before he jumped on a bus, I launched myself out of the door into torrential rain wearing a thin pair of socks and proceeded to run after him down the street begging him to return. He batted me off like an annoying fly, never spoke to me again, and I scuttled home with soaking wet feet and great big tears rolling down my face, mixed with mascara and rain. It wasn't pretty.

I had moments like this in the weeks after I parted company with alcohol. I desperately craved the magic wand which would blot out any negative feelings, and the rush of false confidence that used to make me feel sexy and vivacious no matter where I was and whose presence I was in. Without alcohol I felt drab and uninteresting and pointless. But still I hung on because the alternative was worse – to return to Mr Unsuitable and a life of traumatic ups and downs, emotional upsets and a whole lot of heartache.

It is worth remembering that the human brain is fully capable of physically rewiring itself, given enough time to do so. Allowing sufficient time for this to happen means not drinking at all, as even the odd glass or night of alcoholic indulgence will undo (or at least drastically slow down the process) the neurological alterations that have been taking place unnoticed in your grey matter ever since you decided to ditch the booze.

It is inevitable that when you first cut alcohol out of your life you will have the odd or perhaps intensely frequent, depending on your level of addiction and consumption, craving for a drink. These thought processes will eventually diminish over time but it is important to remember at the outset that our brains need a fairly substantial length of time to become rewired.

Neurological pathways lie behind our habits, the neuroplasticity of our grey matter meaning we are forever altering of our brain's structure and function, which in turn affects the habits we employ and our general behaviour. In simple terms, the more you tread a particular path of your neural network, the stronger and apparently 'natural' the associated behaviour will become.

'Practice makes perfect' is not simply a throwaway maxim – it is neurological fact.

Breaking a long-standing habit or addiction can take time which can be frustrating. As the weeks drag by and you find yourself experiencing longing and desirous thoughts about the cold, crisp taste of Chardonnay on a summer's evening, it can feel as though you will never successfully move forward and think differently. But you will – eventually. The key to this change in your thinking patterns occurring is to make a commitment to sobriety.

If you were to set out as a newly-wed with the idea lurking somewhere in your mind that if everything goes to pot then you can bale out and find a replacement partner, your marriage would more than likely fail. The reason marriage works and lasts for many decades (for a large number of people at least) is because when they declare their vows they really mean them, and crucially they remember them during the tough times.

'To have and to hold, from this day forward, for better, for worse, for richer, for poorer, in sickness and in health, to love and to cherish, 'till death do us part. And hereto I pledge you my faithfulness.'

People often ask me how I have managed to maintain sobriety and the reason, quite simply, is that I made a commitment to never drinking alcohol again. I decided to live without alcohol no matter what life throws at me. An old friend of mine quit drinking alcohol and in the early weeks whenever she had a craving would ask herself this; 'Would a glass of wine make this situation better?' Obviously the answer was always no and thus she maintained her daily existence without booze.

Alcohol depresses the central nervous system – it can cause or exacerbate existing problems of depression and anxiety. Heavy and regular drinking can make it difficult to cope with small problems in life that shouldn't be so much of an issue. However, the short-term 'lift' to our sense of wellbeing (despite being false and impossible to maintain) can fool us into believing that alcohol is actually helping us to feel better. The simple truth is it does not make us feel better and ultimately alcohol can cause a whole multitude of mental health problems which make dealing with anything in life harder than it would otherwise be, should we abstain from alcohol.

The early weeks and months of living alcohol-free can be testing to say the least. Just as the initial period of singledom following the break-up of a long relationship can find you fighting the urge to text or phone your ex-partner and ask him to come over and give you a cuddle, so the first few weeks of sobriety will throw up many occasions when you are desperate to run up to the shop and buy in some wine. Resist! It is this early period that will lay the foundations for a long-term commitment to sobriety – give it a chance; give yourself a chance. Concentrate on all the amazing aspects of your character that you have been covering up with alcohol for so long.

Reading the posts and comments on Soberistas.com throws up a whole host of brilliant and positive consequences which come about as a result of people ending their long-lasting dependencies on alcohol. Members of the site write about how their relationships with spouses and children have improved, how they have lost weight and become more focused on eating healthily, about new fitness goals and the newly discovered pleasures of running, dance classes, or visiting a gym. These outward differences seen in those who have begun to live alcohol-free are only the tip of the iceberg; for many, the major changes following the decision to stop drinking are to be found in their personality.

I continue to surprise myself with regards to my newfound ability to cope in stressful situations, to not work myself into a frenzy over some trivial nonsense but to process things in a measured and calm fashion and subsequently come up with a good, workable solution, to think first before opening my mouth, to have confidence in my beliefs and to have the passion and drive to continually aim higher in many aspects of my life.

Living life as a drinker for me was akin to bobbing along, head barely showing above the surface of a murky pond. It was as though I was caught in a restrictive, suffocating quagmire of low self-esteem and no confidence, with zero desire to improve myself and my life. I simply existed, trapped by the endless negativity that alcohol-dependency casts over those it ensnares.

By reading this book, you have already demonstrated an interest in living alcohol-free. The thought of leaving behind the destructive and regrettable consequences of regular and heavy alcohol consumption has been there in your mind, poked its face up and said a quiet 'hello' to make its presence felt. In order to act upon this thought, it is vital that you establish the reasons why you are experiencing even the tiniest of desires to cut alcohol out of your life and get things back on track.

Try writing the reasons down and keeping the list safe to reread whenever you need a reminder. Include absolutely everything; the shame you have felt, the feelings of remorse and regret for silly drunken actions that you never meant once you'd sobered up and for which you have struggled so hard to forgive yourself, how rough you look in the mornings post-drinking, how much rubbish you feel compelled to eat when hungover resulting in a constant failure to stick to diet or fitness regimes, the damage you may be doing to your body in the long-term, drunken arguments, lack of patience with your children, repeated inability to find the energy to change an unwanted situation, be it your job or financial situation or relationship that you feel ran its course years ago – all of these consequences of heavy drinking are behind the little voice that you occasionally hear whispering to you "You must stop drinking."

Now remind yourself of this – if you continue to drink,

things will not change. Ever. It is crucial that you wrap your head around this notion because it is the key to unearthing the level of commitment required for real change. In order to make the promise to yourself that you will live alcohol-free you must truly want to change your life and if that is the case, then you must recognise that the negative roller-coaster to which you have been clinging all these years can only be brought to a standstill if you alter the path you are currently following. If you are happy with your life, keep everything pretty constant; if you hate your life, you need to enact change and you will find it impossible to bring about that change if you are regularly drinking more than the recommended amount of alcohol.

The equation is simple – Love life; maintain the status quo. Hate life; something major has to change. The key piece of advice with regards to this sum is that you will struggle to change anything major in your life if you continue to drink. You may attempt to moderate your alcohol consumption but if you have an emotional dependency on this addictive substance you will find it damn near impossible to drink in a controlled fashion; eventually old habits will resurface.

You are now facing a crossroads – continue as you have been and the results will remain the same, or take a completely new path, shedding your old habits like dead skin and looking forward to bigger and brighter things in your future. If you cannot make the commitment you should stop reading now.

If you have made your mind up to take the path to a new life,

CONGRATULATIONS!

You may decide to celebrate your new commitment to sobriety by announcing it to the world on Facebook, throwing a lavish

(AF) party or inviting friends and family round to tell everyone at once thus getting 'it' out in the open. Or you may choose to make a silent promise to yourself, and quietly get on with the business of enjoying life free from the shackles of addiction. Whichever celebration you decide on, be sure to take time out to congratulate yourself on this decision; the old self-hatred, crippling feelings of shame and regret and berating yourself for not having more control are no more. From now on, you are on the up – the mornings of recriminations and worry have come to an end and the future holds some or all of the following for you to look forward to;

Learning who you are minus the cloak of alcohol, rebuilding your confidence and self-esteem, putting real effort into exciting new projects and seeing results, enjoying guilt-free quality time with your friends and family, looking fresher and younger, losing weight, better quality sleep, and feeling more in control of you and your life.

Your choice to devote yourself to sobriety is one which you will thank yourself for, both in the near future and in the longer term of your life. Making the decision to live alcohol-free is something of which you should be very proud; this valuable lifestyle choice could help you to finally realise your full potential.

CHAPTER THREE

The Honeymoon Period

You are now enjoying your first taste of freedom following a dependency on alcohol which is likely to have caused you no end of trouble. The sense of liberation which arises from knowing that you will never again wake up suffering a complete memory blackout of the previous night's events, nor waste an entire weekend struggling to cope with a debilitating hangover, can be enough to plaster a huge smile on your face from ear to ear.

In the early days, you may be wondering what on earth you were so terrified of as you feel better, look better, and have so much energy that you don't know what to do with it all. Below is an extract from the Soberistas blog which details my personal experience of this first stage of sobriety;

'As an alcohol-dependent person who had felt terribly out of control of her own life for many, many years, the first couple of weeks of living as a non-drinker were a breath of fresh air. The joy of waking up each day and not immediately running through a mental checklist of who I had insulted/let down/hurt the night before was beyond compare. I literally jumped out of bed each day, a massive weight of anxiety removed from around my neck. Gone were the fears of developing breast cancer or dying of liver failure; the dreaded guilt and shame that

I suffered as a result of doing something stupid and/or irresponsible when under the influence had vanished – I felt free as a bird. Going out socially was a wonderful experience, as previously I had always felt butterflies in my stomach as I feared how the night ahead would unfold, never knowing how drunk I would get and where that state of mind would take me. Instead I knew that I was finally calling the shots – I would decide who to talk to, what I said, whether or not I chatted someone up/allowed myself to be chatted up; this was me, and not that idiot who I became after too much wine.'

Just as your real-life honeymoon should be defined by your head-over-heels love for each other with none of the nerve-grating annoyances that may reveal themselves further down the line, for many people this period of newly adopted sobriety is a happy and fairly easy period of adjustment.

Breaking free from a dependency on alcohol is akin to escaping from a self-built prison; you suddenly realise that you've been incarcerated for years although while trapped in the cycle of addiction you had no idea that you were effectively restricted behind bars. Most of your thoughts, actions, the social events you attend, the dinner parties, how you choose to spend your leisure time and even sexual encounters have most probably occurred while under the influence of, or recovering from the effects of, alcohol. Much of your life was more than likely planned around opportunities to drink without you even noticing.

With hindsight I recognise that in my past drinking life I arranged for friends to come round for a dinner or nibbles purely because it presented the perfect occasion to get drunk. That's what we do at such events isn't it? Friends arrive at your door bearing multiple bottles of wine and the expectation hangs in the air unspoken but mutually agreed – tonight it is OK to get smashed. And smashed I would proceed to become. Every social engagement I entered into involved excess drinking, from attending gigs, festivals, nightclubs, meals in restaurants, children's birthday parties – without exception all ultimately led to an almighty piss-up. I was therefore coached very proficiently in having low expectations of my behaviour and the general outcome of any social function I attended. All would almost always result in me offending someone, acting like an idiot, causing deep upset or hurt to a friend or partner or conking out on the host's settee like a corpse.

My honeymoon period with sobriety was, therefore, a time during which I felt as though I'd rediscovered my ability to breathe. I avoided pubs and socialising with those who I knew had drunkenness forefront in their minds when on a night out. For me this was a sensible option and I would advise you to do the same; it doesn't have to be for ever and there may come a point when you feel entirely comfortable sitting alongside a bunch of drunken monkeys who are propping the bar up and talking mostly rubbish to each other. But certainly in the early period of adjustment to a new life of sobriety I would avoid like the plague anywhere or anyone who may attempt to convince you to return to the prison you have just managed to escape from.

Rather than hiding away at home in fear of temptation, however, aim to obtain your social fix by meeting either non-drinkers or friends who drink but in situations where they aren't drinking, e.g. a coffee in the park, a trip to the cinema/theatre, or a lunch date.

In honesty my feelings towards sobriety were, in the early days, somewhat paradoxical. On the one hand there was blessed relief at the lack of hangovers, the clear head, better sleep, brighter eyes and a sudden ceasing of all regrettable and shameful incidents which had erstwhile occurred several times a week as a result of drinking excessively. On the other side of the coin, I missed my old friend Mr Unsuitable terribly. I craved the excitement and the quick buzz of that first drink; I longed to experience again the fast-track unwinding that comes from a couple of large glasses after a long day. I felt torn in two – part of me was grateful to have finally escaped my prison, the other half was terrified at how on earth I would get on with the rest of my life without alcohol by my side.

There were numerous points in my first weeks without booze when I was overwhelmed with happiness and love for simple things which I had taken for granted for so long. The sun rising over the park while I was out running with the dog, a blossom tree just coming into bloom, sharing a joke with my daughter and hearing her laugh – I felt as though my senses had been heightened and all of a sudden I was feeling things as a real person with all their faculties intact, rather than the hazy, fogged alcohol-obsessed person I had been previously.

Luckily there were no terrible incidents in my life at that time which may have caused me to have a wobble with regards to my commitment to sobriety and my new life. Things ticked along quietly and I largely kept my head down and attempted to focus on all things positive. As long as I was busy and in a reasonably good mood the notion of Pinot Grigio rarely entered my head – only on the odd evening when I was alone with nothing to keep me occupied did my thoughts drift to the cold bottles I knew were sitting up the road in the chiller cabinet of the supermarket.

Despite the fact that at times during this honeymoon period I occasionally missed the excitement of my past love affair with wine, I refused to give into temptation as I had made a solid commitment to sobriety and felt very strongly that nothing good would ever come of my life if I indulged in the short-term hit of an alcohol binge, and that to achieve real change I had to remain alcohol-free. I was thirty-five and a mum who was still trying to scrape her way out of the financial mess brought about by divorce and single-parenthood, and if I drank just one bottle of wine on any given night, it was tantamount to admitting defeat and remaining for ever in that miserable hole I had found myself in. My desire to improve mine and my daughter's lives was huge, and alcohol would only have served as a preventative measure in bettering our situation.

The really positive moments when I appreciated life minus the negativity of alcohol which had pulled me down for so long were moments of true joy and happiness. I will never forget the sunrise I watched while running through the park at 6am with just my dog and a lonely heron, perusing the pond for breakfast, for company, or the times I spent with my daughter when I found myself concentrating on her and what we were doing together one hundred per cent without hankering after my next wine fix and wondering how long I would have to wait until I could pour a glass.

Those moments were little droplets of heaven.

Amidst all of the good times, however, you are bound to feel a whole range of emotions, positive and negative, as you're no longer using the crutch of alcohol to coast along through life's difficulties; now you have to actually cope with feelings and this can be tough, particularly if you have been drowning your emotions for many years. Being upset really hurts without alcohol – although conversely, when you experience real happiness you definitely know about it when you aren't slightly inebriated!

If you enter into the honeymoon period with the following expectations then you should be prepared to cushion yourself in order to remain true to your commitment (remember that sobriety is just like a real person in that your relationship will involve highs and lows and many mediocre moments in between – the trick is to know you will endeavour to honour your promise, no matter what);

1)   You will probably experience moments of real exhilaration and overwhelming happiness in the early period of sobriety as your body and mind begin to absorb your surroundings free from the dense fog that alcohol wrapped around your being.

2)   Your body has been used to absorbing an addictive substance for quite some time and therefore you will suffer pangs and cravings during the honeymoon period as you become physically and mentally readjusted to life without alcohol.

3)   Your self-esteem has a long way to go to repair itself after the effects and consequences of regular alcohol abuse will have taken their toll. At times you will possibly feel unsure and vulnerable and this will most likely make you REALLY want a drink – try to recognise this inner voice as Mr Unsuitable who is trying desperately to win you back – he never thought you'd have the balls to leave and now that you have he doesn't like it one bit. Make it obvious that you mean business; now is the time to build your confidence back up, and learning to turn down this pest's advances will help give you a major boost in this area!

4)   You may encounter a strong sense of boredom in the

evenings and especially at the weekend – any long-standing habit takes a while to break but you can help yourself by planning a distraction to keep your mind elsewhere during those occasions when you might become fidgety for wine; playing a board game, taking up a hobby, partaking in a sport, or catching up with films that have been on your 'to watch' list for ages but you somehow repeatedly forgot about them in favour of drinking wine. These are all possible ideas, but anything that helps you avoid missing alcohol by keeping your mind and headspace otherwise engaged is perfect.

Armed with a little forethought and preparation, you should be able to enjoy your honeymoon period of sobriety, relishing the freedom from your wine-obsessed thinking patterns. Sooner or later though, you will quite probably encounter a backlash of desire to return to your old ways as the rose-tinted glasses come out and your nostalgic view of hazy, drunken days gone by take on a whole new (and totally edited by Mr Unsuitable himself!) look. As you move into this next phase of beating your alcohol dependency, you may be asking yourself this question – 'OMG have I done the right thing?'

CHAPTER FOUR

OMG, have I done the right thing?

Whether in the days, weeks, or months following your decision to stop drinking, there will likely be occasions when you seriously question your decision to live an alcohol-free life. In my experience there are two major thinking processes behind this pervasive doubt; the rosé-tinted spectacles, and well-meaning friends and family.

Rosé-Tinted Spectacles

If you think back to any love affair in which you have argued with your partner you should be able to remember the phenomenon that is the rosé-tinted glasses; you've had an almighty row, you KNOW you are in the right and have told your erstwhile beloved exactly what you think of them, you flounce out of the door and promise yourself that this is it – no more excuses, no more giving in. The time has come when you will stand resolute to everything you believe in and that you've said. A few hours/days pass, you miss the good times and have a constant memory playback in your head featuring only the highlights; the laughter in the rain, the flowers he bought you when you were ill, the beautiful restaurant he whisked you to for your last anniversary ... and you pick up the phone and make contact.

Now replace this human lover with your old adversary, alcohol. As the period of sobriety has lost some of its novelty sheen you may have begun to think longingly about the 'good times.' Sipping cold white wine in a pub garden decorated with dazzling hanging baskets and the tinkling sound of gay laughter while all around you are having a jolly good time (because they are drinking alcohol of course), the romantic nights after the kids have been put to bed and you and hubby are snuggled up in front of the TV with a bottle of red and a spot of catch-up viewing to enjoy, lingering Sunday roasts with friends who share your love of good food and fine wines – it all seems so wonderful when you think back and the dreaded fear begins to take hold; will life ever be the same again now that you've ditched alcohol?

The issue of denial is worth a mention at this juncture. 'Being in denial' is not something that only happens to hard-core alcohol-addicted people who pour vodka over their cornflakes; denial is present in anyone who is emotionally, mentally, or physically dependent on any substance and who refuses to see that this is the case.

I used to regularly drink at least one bottle of wine a night and approximately tripled my intake over the weekends when my daughter was away at her dad's house. Years ago I picked bottles that I fancied after surveying the label and reading the bumph on the back, and whichever I believed would best suit the meal I was planning on cooking. As time went on, however, my choice of wine was made on a) strength of alcohol by volume (% ABV) and/or b) whichever bottle was subject to the best price deal thus enabling me to buy it in greater quantities.

Clearly this was due to the fact that as the years passed by I yearned after a greater hit and was thus making my wine selections based on my need to fulfil that craving, rather than to bolster the pretence of my being a connoisseur and caring which grape went with what food flavours. My insistence on cooking elaborate meals to accompany the wine I bought (note that the pairing of food and wine really should be in reverse – i.e. the wine should be chosen to accompany the food) was because I was in denial. I wanted to believe that I was a sophisticated young woman who was gradually developing her knowledge of wines and becoming something of an expert, rather than an alcohol-dependent manic depressive who was struggling to get through the evenings without clutching a large glass of vino. The latter just doesn't sound so refined.

During my early weeks of sobriety I experienced such strong and intense waves of denial that I effectively rewrote my personal history in order to attempt to convince myself that a reunion with alcohol was a must. The evenings with friends which in reality had almost always concluded with somebody pouring me semi-conscious into a taxi, in which I was then driven home, entirely trusting that a complete stranger taking me across town in the middle of the night wouldn't rape or rob me, ceased to exist in my memory. Instead I recalled wonderful sun-drenched afternoons spent sipping champagne, laughing together with friends as the sun slowly sank and we remained long into the night smoking and drinking and being convivial. This version always saw me looking pretty in a beautiful summery dress, with none of the slipped features and heavy eyelids that would actually come about after a prolonged session of drinking.

Romantic evenings in restaurants during which I was interesting, captivating, sexy, and desirable replaced the true instances when I had gone out for a meal with a partner, drank wine as though my life depended on it, grown horribly drunk and engineered an argument for no apparent reason, perhaps flirted (or worse) with a total stranger in front of my then boyfriend's eyes and eventually been bundled into a cab and dumped into bed once home to sleep it off.

Denial is cunning and insidious and its voice is well-disguised to sound like the real you.

Selective memory is a wonderful tool used by the addictive mind of someone who has not quite shaken the tenacious hold of an alcohol dependency. In addition to rewriting the past in order to ameliorate a multitude of drunken disastrous incidents, cherry-picking only the 'good times' is a common method employed by Mr Unsuitable to try and convince your rational self that next time will be different – next time you will be able to drink in control and with none of the awful repercussions that have manifested in the aftermath of previous binge-drinking sessions. Just as is the case when harbouring a secret fancy to rekindle the flame of an old (repeatedly destructive) relationship, the devil on your shoulder will pull every trick out of the book in order to keep you close to his chest.

The voice which tells you that 'next time will be different' is one to be ignored at all costs. If you have years of destructive drinking patterns behind you, if you perpetually fail to recognise mid-drinking session when you have had 'enough,' if you repeatedly consume way above the government guidelines of fourteen units of alcohol per week for women or twenty-one for men, if you can relate to waking up to feelings of shame and regret following a heavy alcohol binge the night before, and if you have made it this far into reading this book, then chances are the voice you are hearing telling you that 'next time will be different' is lying.

51

The '*next time will be different*' message is being directed at the real you by your dependence upon alcohol. It is the voice of the unsuitable partner who you have finally managed to leave and who is now begging for one more chance as this time things have changed – he has changed. He appreciates you and sees where he went wrong during your relationship; he's realised his behaviour must alter. He is ready to commit to you, to stop letting you down and lying, to quit cheating on you with other people, to prioritise you and your needs and to listen to you when you need him. He is persuasive and comes bearing flowers and chocolates. He looks good too as he's lost some of the weight he has gained recently and had a haircut. You are tempted to believe him when he says that things will be different. You really want to have faith in him because a big part of you just wants to take the easy way, avoiding the arduous and rocky road of singledom and all its associated self-discovery and emotional challenges. Staying the same can be less frightening than stepping into the unknown – even though 'the same' has caused you huge problems for a long time.

Making a commitment to sobriety means the selection of a potentially treacherous path – for a while at least. The unearthing of the real you and the inevitable task of coping with negative events and situations without the prop of alcohol will necessarily be tough to begin with. However, the difficulties faced during the first few months of sobriety will help you develop as a person and to grow much stronger so that ultimately you won't need alcohol to cope when things hit the fan. You will manage just fine with your natural faculties; in fact you'll manage a whole lot better than you ever did with Mr Unsuitable dragging you down.

The short-term fix of sinking a bottle of plonk, or whatever was your poison, will NOT grant you long-term happiness – guaranteed. The only way you can achieve that is to determine to navigate your way through the initial challenges that life throws at you alcohol-free, thus building up your inner emotional strength. When you come out the other side it will be easy as pie to ignore the 'this time will be different' voice – you'll be able to do it while walking down the wine aisle of Tesco; I know because I do.

Well-Meaning Friends & Family

'*OMG have I done the right thing?*' is a question which you may ask yourself as a result of well-meaning friends and family attempting to persuade you that you never had a drink problem and that your stated intention to live the rest of your days alcohol-free is a teensy bit of an overreaction. Alternatively you may have been leading such a destructive existence as a result of your heavy alcohol consumption that friends and family are blissfully relieved that you've finally resolved to quit; if the latter is applicable to you, then you may wish to skip the following section of the book.

One of the hardest aspects of choosing to adopt a sober lifestyle is coming to the realisation in the first instance that you do have a problem with alcohol. We live in a world which is filled with glamorous imagery of beautiful people sipping boozy beverages without giving it a second thought, a world in which a complimentary drink upon arrival at a hotel or in business class of an aeroplane is routinely presented as a selection of something alcoholic, a world which considers it appropriate to become inebriated at birthdays, weddings, christenings, anniversaries, Christmases, and other family get-togethers. Letting your hair down, having a laugh, winding down – these are all expressions that are associated with the excessive consumption of alcohol and nowhere is this more prevalent than in the UK (as far as I can tell). Booze is ubiquitous in Western culture.

Therefore announcing to your nearest and dearest that you no longer plan to partake in such drunken merriment can be a daunting prospect. On Soberistas.com, I commonly read discussion posts written by women whose husbands have professed a major disappointment in the fact that their wives have decided they won't be guzzling booze with them all weekend any more and will from now on be embarking on new and more productive pastimes instead. For a couple whose marriage has been built on a foundation of alcohol, from the first date, past the boozy initial sexual encounter and onto the alcohol-fuelled wedding, before finally settling into nights sitting in front of the TV, wine to hand after the kids have fallen asleep in an effort to unwind together, alcohol plays a massive role in life. One party of the relationship backing out of this unspoken, unwritten rule of engagement of alcohol always being present and effectively amounting to a third person in the marriage, can be terrifying to the still-drinking spouse.

Fears over the drying up of conversational topics, how to go about the act of sex minus the multiple glasses of mental and emotional lubrication beforehand, a real sense of dread regarding socialising with other couples while one person remains stone-cold sober and the rest of the group slowly becomes sloshed; these are all possible concerns which may prompt your alcohol-consuming partner to berate your decision to stop drinking.

A fact of life is that simply because there are elements of good in something, this is not, in itself, sufficient enough reason to continue to ignore all its negatives. If you were married to someone who beat you up and verbally assaulted you approximately once or twice a month but for the remainder of the time was attentive and loving and wonderful, would these positives erase the terrible abuse? Of course they wouldn't.

We can sometimes have a good time while drinking alcohol. If you are regularly engaged in destructive drinking patterns then it is more probable that consuming alcohol will result in a series of not-so-pleasant outcomes, but even so, there will likely be the odd night out here and there when you do manage to rein it in, you are in the company of someone who you genuinely like (with or without the booze – we'll come to that later) and therefore enjoy socialising with him/her and for whatever serendipitous reasoning the alcohol does not result in you passing out/throwing up/acting inappropriately/degrading yourself/behaving thoroughly irresponsibly – delete as appropriate. We would be pretending if we said that such drinking events did not occur.

The crucial point to grasp from this acknowledgement, however, is that the occasional trouble-free evening of boozing is not evidence of the fact that you might NOT have a problem with alcohol. The odd nightmare-free evening of drinking is down to a fluke, a surprising and happy blip in a landscape of alcohol-fuelled horrors. Wrap your head around this fact and stick to your guns in reminding yourself of the truth when faced with the temptation to drink alcohol; the occasional night of drinking which doesn't end in disaster is NOT evidence that you will no longer endure terrible repercussions because of the alcohol you drink; it is a pleasant one-off. Chances are that if you pick up where you left off and waltz back to the land of boozing, sooner or later you will end up in exactly the same place that you so desperately wanted to escape from in the first place.

It took me twenty long years to reach this acceptance of my drinking behaviour but when the penny eventually dropped it landed with a resounding crash. If I begin drinking again there will come a time, maybe in a week, a month, or a year, when I will go bananas with wine. I will down the stuff like I have been dehydrated in a desert for days on end, pour glass after glass as though terrified that it will be taken away from me and so I must therefore consume it as quickly as possible, ultimately seeking out every bottle or can of alcoholic liquid in my near vicinity and drinking the whole damn lot until I pass out. That's me, and it always will be.

Friends and family who do not have the same destructive relationship with booze as you do will not be able to empathise with the very dark lows you have endured as a result of your inability to stop drinking once you have begun. The deep sense of shame and the cold, far-reaching hand of self-loathing that acts as a barrier to emotional strength, thus making it so hard to escape the cycle of drinking and regret, are almost impossible to appreciate if you have never suffered from addiction. For the addiction-free friend or partner, the ability to put a cork in it when they have had enough is down to a simple decision that everyone should be equipped to make, just as they do and every other 'responsible drinker' does. They will therefore perceive your choice to live alcohol-free as unnecessary and over-the-top when in their mind you could very easily just moderate your alcohol consumption by learning to recognise your own limit.

You, however, know that you cannot do this. It is you who has endured all the destructive consequences of heavy drinking for so long, coming to realise that you never know when enough is enough, that you fail to recognise when you are becoming drunk and out-of-control, and that you are sick to death of staring at a reflection in the mirror that you despise.

Many people do not like the idea of giving up drinking alcohol and particularly if it hasn't caused them too much anguish they will most likely not see why they should. Such people may consider your decision to stop drinking as one which throws their own consumption into the spotlight, and this is something which could result in a degree of discomfort for them.

None of this is of any concern to you, however. There is only one person on the planet who truly knows how much you've suffered at the hands of this thoroughly destructive relationship with a lover hell bent on sabotaging your future happiness, and that person is you. Believing in something is about having the courage to stand true to those beliefs in the face of criticism or attempts to persuade you to walk a different path from those around you. Having faith in something means grabbing onto all the reasons why you made this choice in the first place and hanging onto them for dear life – do not let well-meaning friends and family who may feel as though their own drinking is being criticised or placed under threat as a direct result of your sobriety tempt you back into a relationship which has caused you such abject misery and pain. This is a matter of self-preservation.

As a smoker I worried almost constantly about my habit causing the development of breast cancer, or any other cancer for that matter. At night I would often lie alone in bed feeling for the lumps I felt certain were growing silently all over my body as manifestations of the malignant disease I had induced by puffing away on so many Marlboro Lights. Conversely, my

57

worries all but vanished when I was in the company of other smokers. Why was this?

'Groupthink' is a construct of social psychology which denotes the actions of people who behave in a deviant way as a result of a desire to conform and a sense of loyalty to the group of which they are a member. Well known examples of groupthink include the atrocities carried out by American soldiers against civilians during the Vietnam War. Obviously smoking and heavy drinking are not in the same league of wrongdoing as murder and rape, but the same mental processes are at work when we reassure ourselves that something which we know is bad is really OK, simply because we are in the company of other people who are carrying out the same dangerous/immoral activity and are seemingly unperturbed by it.

Consider the huddles of smokers to be found outside any office block up and down the country at intervals throughout the day. In this day and age of uber-awareness regarding the dangers of smoking, lone smokers can be made to feel something of a pariah as their habit is accepted in fewer and fewer public places with each passing year. Put those same smokers with other smokers (for instance, outside the office building) and their mood is instantly transformed to something akin to pride – the cigarette has once again become a badge of honour, a symbol of defiance against the non-smoking killjoys.

Groupthink is of relevance to the consumption of alcohol too. If you consider the people who you socialise with, chances are they too 'enjoy a drink' and are prone to the odd (or frequent) bout of exceptionally heavy alcohol consumption leading to drunkenness. Such behaviour feels acceptable when we are in the company of others doing the same, and this can be a major reason behind the fact that people with a problematic dependency on alcohol can take years to arrive at the conclusion that their habit is unhealthy and destructive; when all around you are losing their heads (to paraphrase Rudyard Kipling) it is easy to feel unconcerned that you are losing yours.

In order to successfully conquer the temptation that may be placed before you by well-meaning friends and family despite you informing them that you have decided to quit drinking alcohol, it is imperative that you take on board the above. Try to remove yourself psychologically from your drinking circle of friends where booze is concerned – just because they have shown no worries about their alcohol consumption and the associated mental and physical health risks, this does not mean there aren't any.

If you have felt anxiety with regards to the amount of alcohol you drink to the degree that you would like to live without it, then most probably you are drinking too much. This is for you to decide and nobody else. Do not let other people's dependencies on alcohol influence your decision as to whether to continue drinking it or not. In the end, this is your life and you who must listen to the thoughts playing out in your head.

As a person who lives free of the constraints of alcohol, you will soon develop an acute sense of who you are and what you want from life. This self-awareness may not be present currently as alcohol robs you of this valuable life skill but it will grow over time just as soon as you allow it to flourish minus the smothering nature of alcohol. As the weeks go on, sticking to your belief that you are better off without alcohol will become easier – in these early days try and keep the faith that you do know best, no matter what anyone else tells you.

CHAPTER FIVE

Building the Lasting Relationship

Hopefully by now you will be feeling more confident in the decision you have made to end your relationship with Mr Unsuitable and happy to settle into a union with sobriety. Do not underestimate the amount of adjusting you will have to do before you become accustomed to living alcohol-free; this will not happen overnight.

Just as with marriage or a long-term relationship, you must accept in your mind that you have made a commitment to sobriety and are therefore prepared to stick to your new lifestyle through thick and thin. Giving up smoking would be impossible if every person who tried rushed out to buy a packet of fags every time they encountered a little difficulty in life.

Life is difficult – it is also wonderful and rewarding and exciting, but nobody's life comes minus the challenges. I hit the bottle particularly hard in the aftermath of my divorce which happened when I was just twenty-seven. I clearly remember hearing the voice of Mr Unsuitable telling me in no uncertain terms that I deserved wine; I was going through a nightmarish time and I absolutely had the right to drink as much as I wanted to get me through the night. And I did have that right, but that doesn't mean it was the correct path to take. My general attitude around that time was probably best described as 'bloody-minded' and I was firmly in the self-destruct camp of break-up recovery.

So, would I do things differently now with the benefit of hindsight? Yes, I think I probably would, and here's why.

Being a mum is hard work, and being a single mum is very hard work. In addition we live in a society which places aesthetic beauty, particularly in females, at a very high value – maybe the highest. When celebrities become mothers we are not interested in discovering whether they are enjoying the experience and if they are finding it difficult or tiring. No, what we want to know is whether they have shrunk back into their size ten jeans yet and if there are any horrific wobbly belly shots of them wearing a bikini to gawp over.

There are virtually no older models employed in the advertisement of beauty products and those that are tend to be slim, glamorous, and rather more attractive than your average woman on the street. Being a mum and struggling to deal with the associated drooping body parts, stretch marks, under-eye bags and dark circles, exhaustion, extra weight that is difficult to shift, and on top of all that coping with the children themselves, running a house, maintaining a relationship (or being lonely as a result of having no relationship), and for many, going to work, takes its toll on our self-confidence.

Going through all of the above while simultaneously being bombarded by air-brushed imagery of stunning women who look a million times more beautiful than us mere mortals could ever wish to can induce feelings of low self-worth and debilitated self-esteem. For many women, wine becomes a welcome relief from this cycle of negativity in which we find ourselves all of a sudden in our thirties and forties.

Here's the problem; wine does not eradicate any of the

61

problems we may encounter as a result of growing older and more frazzled after having kids – it exacerbates them. As someone who has had two babies, one aged twenty-three when I was a drinker (albeit stopping temporarily for pregnancy and breastfeeding) and one aged thirty-six as a non-drinker, I have tested out both sides of the coin and there is a palpable difference in both my ability to cope with the demands of motherhood and in my general mental wellbeing.

At twenty-three I had the mind-set of a party animal – my husband and I and our large circle of like-minded friends regularly got together for parties, meals out or at each other's houses, children's birthdays, and shared holidays, and alcohol played a very important part of the whole scene. Looking back it was a time defined by booze and socialising. In contrast my life now is centred on my family and although I go out with friends and my partner and I socialise as a couple, it is not the be all and end all of our existence. I do not drink at all, and my partner rarely drinks (he goes out with friends once or twice a week) and never in the house.

Despite being thirteen years older this time around, I have more patience and energy, and have found that I enjoy every second with my baby with none of the short-temperedness that I remember first time around when, for instance, my eldest daughter wouldn't go to sleep or eat her dinner, or wouldn't stop prattling and asking incessant questions about everything and anything. I see quite clearly now that this lack of patience was because I was usually hungover and tired, or because I was itching for her to go to sleep so I could get downstairs, switch into adult time, and crack the wine open.

Despite running a half-marathon when my first daughter was two years old, I was drinking heavily and regularly all through her childhood. My weight hovered around two stone heavier than I would have liked and I never managed to lose those extra pounds until the depression and anxiety really set in during my marriage break-up (aka the Divorce Diet). Excluding the bursts of false happiness when I was under the influence of alcohol, I look back on a largely unhappy person when I consider myself in my twenties. Drinking excessively on a regular basis resulted in the onset of a range of difficult-to-budge mental and physical negative consequences that I attempted to cope with or forget altogether by consuming yet more wine.

I include the above history because when you enter into the early phase of your commitment to sobriety it is essential that you focus on the positive reasons why you are doing this. Even if you are tempted to cave in when you have had a bad day with the kids, or your partner isn't pulling his weight around the house, or your spare tyre is getting bigger and you haven't the energy or motivation to tackle it, drinking will only alleviate these concerns temporarily and will, in actual fact, make them worse in the long run.

Giving up drinking is, at this stage, a simple trade-off; let go of the short-term 'Mummy's little helper' and accept that there will be an interim period of no man's land, but that if you stay committed and work your way through the challenges that will inevitably present themselves to you during that time, you will come out the other side a million times stronger and without the need to depend emotionally on alcohol.

If you can relate to all or some of the above issues arising from the experiences of motherhood, then reassure yourself constantly through this stage that while it will take some time, many of the negative aspects of life that you may have been attempting to ease with alcohol consumption will eventually disappear without the booze (for instance, general low mood leading to being snappy with the kids and/or your other half, over-eating carbs because of a perpetual hangover, feeling tired and groggy due to poor quality and lack of sleep), and the things that you dislike but cannot change (your height/boob size/mother-in-law) will be much easier to deal with once you have the clarity that an alcohol-free life brings.

I know that I am by no means perfect but rather than allow my insecurities to eat me alive as they did in my drinking days, I am now comfortable in my own skin and the old me who was seriously lacking in confidence is nowhere to be seen – she has been swallowed whole by a determined, positive, energetic, glass-half-full, and sure-footed woman who won't stand for nonsense from anyone. The real you is hiding just beneath the alcoholic fog that you have been living in for such a long time and now is the time to concentrate on bringing her to the fore.

Building the foundations on which to base a lasting commitment to sobriety is essentially something which happens very gradually, just as with a conventional marriage. You need to become accustomed to each other and learn how to act in a whole number of situations that life throws in your joint path.

Socialising is a big issue when you are new to sobriety. As discussed in Chapter Four, we live in a society which considers alcohol consumption, and excessive alcohol consumption at that, to be entirely normal and even expected. If you suddenly announce to your social circle that you no longer partake in drinking you may feel a little left out to begin with. Unfortunately, one of the most noticeable side-effects of becoming a non-drinker is that you are very suddenly made aware of the people in your life who you do not actually like very much.

Alcohol is great as a people-leveller; it tramples down the uniqueness of individuals and casts a homogeneous light across people who are, in sober reality, very different to each other in character. Alcohol, in short, irons out the wrinkles and presents almost everyone as nice people who you can get along with. When you put down the wine you may discover that many of the people you previously thought you enjoyed the company of are in reality self-righteous dullards who bore you rigid.

The upside of this is that you can now choose to spend time with the people who are genuinely the ones you get along with, and you will discover that you have a great time with them sober or drunk – it has always been, with these people, the friendship and things you have in common that have brought about the good times, and not the booze as you probably imagined.

I have written and spoken much about the need to develop new interests in the wake of quitting alcohol. It is essential if you are to maintain your sobriety that you find other things to do with your time than continue to socialise with heavy drinkers in environments that do little to accommodate those who live alcohol-free. When I consider how I spent my free time in my drinking days I see a pattern of engineered opportunities to get drunk masquerading as social occasions arranged for more wholesome reasons. The dinners I organised, Sunday afternoons in a beer garden with friends and our respective children, romantic nights in restaurants – everything I did was done purely in the name of setting a socially acceptable scene in which I could drink and get drunk.

If you remove the alcohol from the social events that I attended as a drinker, I guarantee that the majority of them would have fallen by the wayside. If the people I socialised with had all packed in drinking en masse, my allegiances with them would have frazzled and dried up like a wilting flower in the desert. I liked their company because I enjoyed the fact that they were relaxed about alcohol and enjoyed using it to alter their minds.

When I stopped drinking I knew that my life would necessarily have to change, big time. I was a party girl for twenty years therefore I had a fifth of a century of behavioural norms to undo and rewrite – no mean feat.

Mentally I think I wiped my history for a while; in a subconscious way I ceased to act like me, most likely because I associated the old Lucy with destruction and unhappiness. I craved being someone new, I desperately wanted to feel like one of those people who is seemingly unbothered by alcohol and is happy to do other things with their time; I could see quite clearly that the old me could not be sustained minus the false reality of booze. And so I set about adopting new habits.

Destructive relationships affect the submissive partner in numerous negative ways which help maintain the longevity of the situation. As the dominant partner wields their manipulative and damaging characteristics, the victim in the situation gradually has their confidence and self-esteem eroded resulting in a real belief that they are unworthy of anything better in life. The recipient of all the soul-crushing abuse becomes so lost and unable to perceive their own situation in the harsh light of day that they unwittingly allow the assault on their personality to continue, furthering the destruction of their self-confidence and ultimately committing themselves to a doomed existence.

As someone who has regularly abused alcohol and is new to sobriety, you will more than likely have low self-esteem. In the early days of living alcohol-free you will perhaps experience feelings of doubt and anxiety with regards to the decision you have made to stop drinking – how will you cope without alcohol? Who will you be without the shortcut to boozy party animal that you have relied on for so long? How will you be able to relate to your friends/family/partner minus the alcoholic sheen that has always galvanised your social life?

Try to eliminate all these thoughts and questions from your mind and concentrate instead on just being. The commitment you have made to sobriety is a big one – a positive one yes, but a biggie nonetheless. Things will change, YOU will change and ultimately the changes that occur will make you happier and better able to cope with life and all that it throws at you but these changes won't happen overnight and you need to allow yourself time to adjust to the new you.

You can make life easier for yourself by engaging in pastimes that keep you busy but don't demand masses of brainpower – knitting, cooking, or going for countryside walks are all excellent for taking you away from the mental danger zone of boredom; when you are bored you are much more likely to feel the urge to fall back into old habits so put into place some damage limitation and prevent the boredom from arising in the first place. When I first stopped drinking I read an awful lot, ran every day, and began to meditate, all of which helped see me through the first few itchy weeks.

Entering into a marriage with sobriety will prove to be good for you so believe in this decision you have made – there are no negatives to be found in a lifestyle choice that will restore your confidence, self-esteem, and happiness while simultaneously eradicating depression, low sense of self-worth, and anxiety or panic attacks. In addition to these positives you will also enjoy having more money and improved physical health and wellbeing – what's not to love?

It is vital to remind yourself, however, that in the early weeks and months of sobriety the insidious voice of Mr Unsuitable, your very own Daniel Cleaver, will attempt to sway you on occasion back to the world of boozing. As you grow in mental strength it will become easier to ignore his persuasive tones but there is no doubt that you will occasionally encounter episodes in which it is almost impossible to resist one last fling with alcohol. Hearing this voice is not evidence that you have done the wrong thing in committing to an alcohol-free life – it is simply the determined and stubborn sound of persistence personified, Mr Unsuitable, desperate to not let you escape from his clutches. Learn to recognise this voice as the alcohol talking and enjoy the sensation of sticking up for yourself, of finding the strength to say no and of knowing you are acquiring a degree of gumption.

Life will change immeasurably for you as a non-drinker but rather than focusing on the elements which you imagine will now be missing, concentrate instead on what you will gain as a result of taking the incredibly strong and positive step to live the rest of your life free from alcohol; you will finally discover who you truly are and recognise your likes and dislikes, you could develop an interest in something creative that you excel at, your relationships will improve as your patience and understanding increase, you will look better and so you'll notice increased self-esteem and confidence, you will finally be able to believe in yourself, and this alone could prove to be the catalyst for dramatic and exciting changes to your whole life.

Stopping drinking opens up your world – it creates opportunity, stretching your horizons beyond the humdrum of the daily grind and the evening 'reward' of a bottle of plonk;

committing to sobriety means far more than simply saying no next time you are offered an alcoholic drink. A commitment to sobriety means learning to know and love the person you are in reality, the one beneath the mask of drunkenness.

Shying away from being a non-drinker will not help your cause. Leaving the booze behind is a decision of which you should be proud – look how many people bumble through their lives spending half of it in a drunken haze and never achieving their potential. If you take the challenging but ultimately life-enhancing step to quit drinking alcohol, you should feel enormously proud of yourself. Hold your head up high and enjoy the knowledge that life will now begin properly for you, and that the mornings of recriminations and self-loathing will be no more. Now is the time to start living, so enjoy it and banish all sense of shame and embarrassment. YOU have just taken control, so pat yourself on the back and begin to enjoy the feeling of liking the person you are for a change.

Attempting to flit in and out of a marriage would never result in a lasting and happy romantic union, just as hoping to manage an addiction to cigarettes without actually giving up is wholly unrealistic, but for a multitude of reasons people often toy with the notion that they can terminate their problematic drinking behaviour by simply imposing a few rules here and there and without actually committing to full time sobriety. In my experience, these efforts to control or moderate alcohol consumption do not work for people who have persistently displayed an inability to drink within reasonable limits. Now is the time to accept that if you want change then the only real way to obtain this is by committing to a sober life, and the best way to assure you stick to your intentions is by adopting a very positive approach to your new alcohol-free existence.

In quitting drinking alcohol, you are not denying yourself anything – you are giving yourself the gift of a life lived in the real world. Take pleasure in waking up free from hangovers and regrets, enjoy knowing that you are doing your best for your family and for yourself, remind yourself of all the benefits, physical and mental, of not drinking alcohol which is a toxic and addictive substance that erodes all sense of who you really are. Sobriety is about making a positive change and setting out on a journey of self-discovery and awareness; get rid of the idea that being a non-drinker equates to missing out on life and replace this thought with the fact that ditching booze will make your life manageable once again, and will restore a degree of calm to everyday living.

Women are often left feeling powerless and put upon in our society, overloaded with childcare responsibilities, caring for other family members, carrying out the lion's share of the housework, forced to work part-time in an underpaid role as a result of taking time out to have and raise children, and doing all of the above while frequently being under-appreciated by those around them. Women can become accustomed to living in a world in which they perceive themselves to have little control over external factors. The heavy consumption of alcohol exacerbates this sense of powerlessness whereas conversely, making the decision to put an end to the relentless cycle of drunkenness, regrets, self-loathing, depression, and anxiety sparks a positive chain reaction based on the recognition that YOU are, in actual fact, the one who calls the shots in your life.

In this phase of building the solid foundations which will ensure a lasting commitment to sobriety, make a real effort to be kind to yourself. Let go of the old negativity and forget (you can work through your regrets later when you are feeling stronger emotionally) the terrible things you may have done or said while under the influence of alcohol. This is a time to focus on restoring your self-esteem and re-establishing your self-confidence; once those elements of your character are back in place you will be in a great position to stay true to your goal of living free from the shackles of alcohol dependency.

Spend the money that you would once have wasted on booze on beauty treatments, good books, or luxurious food – nurture yourself, and tell yourself repeatedly that yes, you are worth it; feeling good inside is not something that only happens to other people. By eating well, pampering yourself and indulging in enjoyable and relaxing activities that you enjoy (whatever they may be) you are reinforcing the idea that you are of value and worth taking care of. Relish frivolity and self-indulgence and cast aside the negative self-image that you've spent too long fostering. Now is the time to:

a)   Rebuild self-esteem and restore lost confidence
b)   Enjoy the feeling of healthful living
c)   Indulge yourself by taking up a pastime that you enjoy

Abusing alcohol erodes self-esteem and robs you of a sense of purpose. Eliminating this poison from your life is the first step to rediscovering exactly who you are, and to finding out how you wish to spend the rest of your life.

CHAPTER SIX

Are Infidelities Really Worth It?

Ok, here comes the million dollar question – can you learn to manage a destructive relationship with alcohol and occasionally have the odd sneaky tipple without it upsetting the apple cart? In short, the answer is no.

This may not be the answer you were hoping for as the devil on your shoulder has perhaps been calling to you recently to come back for one last fling, but the truth is that the real benefits of living alcohol-free come as a result of complete sobriety and if you have struggled with moderation in the past, it's unlikely that it will come easily to you now, if at all.

I believe there are three key factors related to the issue of whether the odd drink will affect your teetotal aspirations, and they are as follows;

1. Re-establishing self-esteem
2. The journey of self-discovery
3. Avoiding the slippery slope

These three factors are unattainable if you disrupt your commitment to sobriety by indulging in just one night of drinking, and without self-esteem, self-discovery and avoidance of the slippery slope you will find it almost impossible to stay on track and away from dependency upon alcohol and all its associated problems.

Let's look at these three crucial factors individually.

Re-establishing your self-esteem

Getting drunk on a regular basis damages your self-esteem. There are numerous reasons for this but the most obvious are a) you do things while under the influence of alcohol of which you are embarrassed and regretful when you sober up, and these drunken actions gradually erode your belief that you are a nice/good person, because nice/good people wouldn't do or say those things would they? Ergo, you must be a bad person, b) alcohol disrupts the central nervous system, causing anxiety and depression and an increased irritability in mood – these changes to a person's mental state can have a knock-on effect on those around them, further adding to a drinker's low self-esteem as he or she then deems themselves to be a terrible parent/partner/friend (delete as appropriate) owing to the negative way he or she interacts with loved ones, and finally c) alcohol is most definitely not a beautifying potion; one of the clearest signs that we are wreaking havoc on our bodies by drinking is to be found in the tell-tale facial signs visible the morning after a heavy boozing session – the red eye area, puffy face, deathly-white and lacklustre skin are all our bodies' way of screaming 'Don't do this to me! I don't like it!' Add to this the growing spare tyre around the waist and you have the perfect ingredients for zero body confidence. Not looking our best adds to the low feelings of self-worth that are brought about by the heavy consumption of alcohol.

73

Below is an extract from the Soberistas blog which describes the depression I was weighed down with as a drinker and how cutting alcohol out of my life has enabled me to overcome my low moods and get back my self-esteem.

'At my lowest ebb I could barely look another human being in the eye. I stopped caring about the level of harm I was inflicting on my physical self, and conversely I harboured thoughts pertaining to hurting myself and the pointlessness of my life.

For a long time since becoming free of alcohol I haven't experienced any real depression or sadness as my life has tended to go from strength to strength ever since I put down the bottle. But I clearly remember the weighty burden of depression and how it made making even the simplest of decisions a frightening and exhausting task of epic proportions.

This is why it can be so incredibly hard to make the choice to stop drinking – the short term relief from feelings of sadness and depression that can be found in alcohol is so tempting in its false ameliorative quality that to find the strength to rebuff it in your darkest of hours is challenging to say the least. And even if you are aware of the negative repercussions of alcohol, when depressed and consumed by self-loathing it is often the intention to inflict further misery on yourself, as opposed to seeking a way out of your depression and into happiness once again.

The thing with all of the above is that if you can find the motivation to stop drinking while feeling so low, fairly soon you will notice a lift in your mood and will gradually witness the rejuvenation of your self-esteem. And when this happens, you will no longer have the intense desire to hurt yourself, rather the opposite will be true; you will want to look after yourself and live a happy existence. In not much time at all, the negative blinkers will fall by the wayside and the world will open up to you as a place filled with possibilities and potential, the restrictive, bleak future that you had mapped out for yourself fading into nothingness.'

After quitting drinking alcohol I would estimate that it took approximately a year for me to restore fully my much damaged self-esteem. For twenty years I had repeatedly piled on the negative, the stupid, the irresponsible, the terrible, and the majorly regrettable incidents to my already fragile levels of confidence and the result was a weak person who would crumble at the slightest sign of a problem, had absolutely no self-belief, and was riddled with self-loathing. Every time I drank and lost control I would act in ways that were so out of character, embarrassing or degrading to me, and wake up the following morning so consumed by self-hatred that I couldn't bear to look in the mirror. My damaged state of mind was as a direct result of drinking, and nothing else.

If you are aware that you cannot control your alcohol consumption unless you abstain completely, then allowing yourself 'the odd night' here and there when you drink is tantamount to compliance with the devil on your shoulder; you are willingly putting yourself at risk of further damage to your self-esteem, which will make it harder and harder to recover from the booze-inflicted harm you are already suffering. You may achieve a night of moderation, but then again you may go wild, drink way too much and find yourself in any one of a number of horrendous situations, none of which you would willingly put yourself in when sober. If you have problems moderating your alcohol intake then risking the occasional dalliance with Mr Unsuitable IS NOT WORTH IT! Chances are you will only wake up in the morning feeling yet more disgusted and annoyed at yourself for your apparent lack of control.

Conversely, affording yourself ample time completely free from drinking in which to recover from the multitude of regrets and embarrassing incidents that have occurred as a result of your alcohol consumption will enable your self-esteem to improve steadily. Imagine never waking up again with that awful sense of dread and self-disgust owing to your drunken behaviour the night before – if for no other reason, that alone is worth never touching alcohol again for (but there are many, many other benefits too, I promise!).

If your self-esteem is low then you may not have the inclination to live a happier and healthier life but the truth is that while ever you continue to drink alcohol on a regular basis, you won't know who you really are or what your full potential is, therefore you aren't capable of making unbiased decisions – for as long as you are drinking alcohol, you are acting as a slave to a drug and not as an autonomous individual. This brings us on to the second important reason why giving in to the odd fling with your old adversary, alcohol, is never a good idea; the journey of self-discovery.

The journey of self-discovery

If you have ever been in a relationship with a controlling partner, or known someone in such an unfortunate situation, you will recognise the characteristics of a person who is unable to act freely and without fear of reproach. A person who is ruled by the repressive persuasions of their abusive or overly-dominant partner gradually loses their sense of individuality and ability to stand up for themselves. Women (because it is usually women who are the victims in a controlling relationship) are commonly transformed from feisty and sure-footed to nervous, won't-say-boo-to-a-goose types without even noticing and after sufficient time has elapsed lose the ability to even decide what clothes to wear without asking their boyfriend or husband's opinion first.

Alcohol, with its insidious and discreet manner, acts in much the same way. Over the years your confidence will grow less but in such a gradual way that you won't be aware it is happening. In social situations you will only feel confident when you have a drink to hand, as the neurotransmitters in your brain are whispering away to you that everything is OK now – good things happen when booze is flowing. Of course this is a falsehood, but you hear this message because alcohol is an addictive substance and therefore your brain is behaving as any other drug addict's brain would; the monster wants to be fed and when you begin to drink you are effectively feeding him.

This endless cycle could continue for your entire life with each day the same as the last; hangover, cravings, pour the wine, feel momentarily better, go to sleep, hangover,r and on and on. When you drink heavily and regularly your world shrinks to fit around your all-important drug of choice, alcohol. Drinking in this way prevents you from growing as a person as your need for more booze outweighs the desire to do anything that doesn't involve drinking. Speaking from personal experience, my weekends as a drinker were engineered from start to finish around wine – inviting people for a meal, meeting up in the pub, picnic in the park (with wine, obviously) – my activities were centred around drinking because I had become mentally and emotionally dependent upon alcohol.

In between drinking I was so hungover or tired that I had neither the energy nor the inclination to involve myself in alternative activities. I had no staying power with regards to any interests that I did manage to take up and so invariably they would fall, one by one, to the wayside because an opportunity to drink would pop up and I would jump at the chance to go and blow my mind on wine again.

In the months leading up to me giving up drinking, I felt a growing sense of panic with regards to the meaningless of my life. I couldn't stand the thought that I might spend the duration of my adult life either drunk or hungover, only to endure the agony in the final days and hours of my life wishing that I could have rewritten my past. In addition, I felt a huge sense of guilt with regards to my lovely daughter, as I knew that my parenting had been less than grand throughout her childhood with much of it defined by my depression, drinking, and moodiness.

These thoughts that I was plagued by were, unbeknownst to me at the time, the foundations being laid for my commitment to sobriety. I wanted more out of life than the pointlessness of drinking – I wanted fulfilment. Self-discovery in my view is not something that can be fully achieved if you are a regular binge-drinker. If you are alcohol-dependent then your world shrinks with your mind encircled by addiction; you are unable to think beyond satisfying those cravings for more booze.

If you want to moderate or control your alcohol consumption then living alcohol-free for the majority of your time but with the odd night of binge-drinking thrown into the mix will not enable you to discover your true self. That only comes from total sobriety, as it is essential that the addictive voice is eradicated completely and you allow YOUR voice to come to the fore unhampered.

Attempts at moderation by alcohol-dependent drinkers result in thought processes that sound something like the following;

> *"I'll only drink at the weekends – Monday to Thursday I will be good, and stay away from the wine."*
>
> *"When I go out, I'll only drink beer – wine is way too strong and I always get hammered, so beer is the way forward. I'll restrict my wine-drinking to home."*
>
> *"I'll have one week every month where I don't drink at all and I'll throw myself into a detox, early nights and fitness for those seven days."*

The outcome of any one of these self-imposed rules (or your own version) is an increase in your obsession with alcohol. The alcohol becomes the forbidden fruit and takes up even more of your thinking time than ever before – your mind goes into overdrive as you attempt to employ willpower as the only ammunition you have in this fight with Mr Unsuitable who is now hell bent on not letting you go. The end result is that you feel deprived, you miss the booze even more than you thought possible and when your period of temporary abstinence is over and done with you are so relieved to get your hands on some wine that you drink three times as much as you set out to.

This point is CRUCIAL to accept if you are seriously looking to get in control of alcohol; the only way to eliminate these thinking patterns is to give up the fight, let go of Mr Unsuitable for good and turn your thoughts to how you will ensure a lasting and solid union with sobriety. Time and time again I read posts on Soberistas.com by women who cannot bear the thought of losing their booze crutch for ever and so attempt to instil a selection of moderating behaviours in their alcohol-dependent minds instead – and time and time again they fail. Alcohol is an addictive substance and when you regularly take any addictive drug, whether it is nicotine, heroin, or alcohol, your mind begins to work overtime in its efforts to ensure you comply with the rules – 'feed me, feed me, feed me' becomes the repetitive drone of the addicted mind.

What you can look forward to as a sober person is a level of clarity that you have most likely forgotten was even possible, an increase in your desire to do new and interesting things in your spare time, a broadening of your mental horizons with a heightened perception of the human experience, and a massive boost to your energy levels as your sleep improves and your body begins to recover from long-term alcohol-abuse.

You will not witness any of the above if you slip in the odd night of binge-drinking; as stated above, all this will do is turn up the volume of your internal booze devil until his voice shouting out for you to drink alcohol becomes impossible to ignore – let it go and move forward in your thinking and your life.

Avoiding the slippery slope

If you have demonstrated repeatedly in the past that you are a person who cannot moderate their alcohol consumption, there is absolutely no reason on earth why this time will be any different. The truth is that once a binge-drinker, always a binge-drinker. On every occasion when you drink to excess, the pathways in your brain that support your emotional and mental dependence on alcohol are reinforced, thus making it harder and harder to break the habit. As soon as you allow yourself one drink the cogs begin to whir, the voice pipes up and Mr Unsuitable is back on your case.

The only solution to this is to always avoid the first drink. The sober mind with its clarity and good intentions may support the notion that one drink is eminently doable and that you are a perfectly normal and able-minded person who can say no after one drink. The problem is that when the first drink slips down, the rational mind becomes tainted with alcohol and the internal booze devil takes over. That's when the trouble begins.

The slippery slope could also arise in the guise of a longer term issue. You may have enjoyed a few weeks off the booze and feel as though things are on the up – the depression has lifted a little, you feel happier and generally more optimistic about life and so you think 'OK, let's give it a go. I will aim to drink no more than a glass of wine on two nights of each week – where's the harm in that?' For anyone who has found themselves in this predicament, the harm is, quite simply, that you have just positioned yourself at the top of a very slippery slope and with each drink you consume you're sliding ever quicker towards the bottom.

Within no time at all there will be an event at which everyone else present is drinking to excess; whether it's a wedding or a birthday or Christmas, sooner or later it's going to happen. As a drinker, albeit a moderate and 'in control' drinker, you will almost certainly become drawn into the mass boozy session around you and drink more than you intended, resulting in the familiar black mornings of recriminations, self-loathing, and remorse. The cycle of negative self-image, drinking to forget your misery, and alcohol-induced depression and anxiety then begins all over again.

You may manage weeks and even months of moderate drinking, but as sure as day is day and night is night, the time will come when, for a plethora of reasons, you'll throw caution to the wind, adopt the 'if you can't beat 'em, join 'em' attitude and drink way more than you set out to.

The slippery slope is only a glass away, for as soon as you allow your mind to become influenced by the external factor of alcohol you cease to act as you. Mr Unsuitable is in charge once again, and with him come all the associated negatives of damaged self-esteem, arguments, blackouts, hangovers, and feeling so exhausted the following day that the entire weekend becomes a write-off.

If you were sick and tired of being involved in a protracted and destructive relationship with a man who perpetually let you down, abused you, cheated on you, and lied, you would, it's to be hoped, eventually break free completely from his control in a desperate bid to find yourself once more and move on with your life. Should you then, having left this awful partner, decide to see him once in a while for the odd night out, nothing serious and no strings attached, you know damn well what would happen – you would be back at square one before you could say 'doormat.' Alcohol is exactly the same and the only true way to resolve the difficulties you have had with it, and to completely free yourself from the tormenting and never-ending chatter of Mr Unsuitable, is to give him the heave-ho for ever.

In this chapter we have examined three very good reasons why a dalliance with alcohol amidst a period of mostly sober living is highly unlikely to prevent you from beating your booze problem on a permanent basis. Although you may fool yourself (or rather, your internal booze demon will try and fool you) that the odd little glass here and there won't hurt, this is simply not true. Becoming sober and happy is not a halfway house; it isn't something that you can achieve if your heart's not in it. Sobriety is a way of life, a commitment, and something that you must own – the prize of sobriety cannot be won by those who try and grab it with one hand while holding a bottle of wine in the other. It simply doesn't work that way.

Putting in place a few rules here and there which limit the type or amount of alcohol that you take is not equal to being in control of it – it is, in actual fact, the opposite. Simply by imposing rules with regards to how frequently you drink or pertaining to the quantity of alcohol that you consume, you are reinforcing the notion that alcohol is in control of you; yet again you are working your life around this drug that has held you in its grip for so long. The ONLY way to be free of the alcohol

> The prize of sobriety cannot be won by those who try and grab it with one hand while holding a bottle of wine in the other. It simply doesn't work that way.

trap is to understand that life will be better without it, and that drinking exacerbates the problems which you have previously imagined were being diminished by the alcohol you drink.

CHAPTER SEVEN

Disagreements and How to Resolve Them

In my experience the doubts that arise over the viability of a long-term commitment to sobriety mostly emerge as a result of the two opposite emotions of joy and abject misery. I never had a problem with the in-between moods, the vast majority of our headspace which is filled with thoughts related to feeling neither ecstatically happy nor woefully sad, but whenever something really bad or really good occurred, that voice would be calling to me to get the wine out (boredom also played a major role in prompting me to drink – the excessive alcohol then preventing me from doing anything worthwhile with my time, resulting in a protraction of my feelings of ennui, and on the vicious cycle would turn).

Summer would burst out from nowhere following long, drawn-out winters and the urge to go and get drunk in a beer garden (or in my own back garden) would be huge. A celebration of any sort, a birthday, graduation, christening, or wedding, or the slightly less life-changing events such as job promotions, having an offer accepted on a house, or someone at work leaving for pastures new – all of these instances would be cause to drink. Such an event happening would provoke a thoroughly unquestioned and innate response of 'let's get absolutely wasted.'

Likewise, negative situations which arose in my life would cause an immediate and undeniable itch for wine; if I ever experienced what I perceived to be a terrible injustice (boyfriend had dumped me, marriage had ended, I didn't get the promotion I had applied for, or I'd had an argument with a friend), off I'd trot to buy some booze from the local supermarket without an iota of worry or doubt that this wasn't the right course of action to take. I had been wronged; ergo I deserved to get hammered.

When suddenly faced with the loss of a loved one, a stressful and emotionally turbulent time such as divorce or redundancy or breaking up with a long-term partner, alcohol can seem to be almost a God-given right, something which you are fully entitled to indulge in given the negative turn your life has just taken. Along with a strong desire to wipe out the pain and thinking related to whatever upset you have recently experienced, there is for many a feeling of wanting to shout 'stuff it!' A two-fingered salute to the world, sent from the safety of your hidey hole, wine in hand and problems forgotten.

These are the times when you are most likely to suffer strong cravings for alcohol, as your body and emotions have become accustomed to meeting your needs by the excessive consumption of booze, and it takes a while to re-programme your mind to respond differently.

For several weeks, maybe months, following my abrupt decision to stop drinking alcohol I also found myself weighed down with a pervading sense of unfairness, that I hadn't really wanted to end my relationship with alcohol but circumstances beyond my control had conspired in such a way as to make it impossible for me to continue. I glared at people sitting outside bars and pubs in the sun, convinced that they were all enjoying this wonderful British pastime of afternoon drinking while here I was, stone cold sober, bored, probably boring, and certainly very pissed off. I failed to see a crucial fact; those people weren't 'allowed' to drink while I was now forbidden to do so – they just hadn't the concerns about alcohol and its negative effects that I had developed over the last few years. They didn't want to stop drinking and didn't see why on earth they should.

Whether or not those concerns aren't present in people who drink alcohol regularly because they do not have a dependency on it or because they do have a dependency on it but are in denial of the fact is an individual matter that varies from person to person. However, rest assured that a number of people who you may witness sitting outside bars and pubs having a jolly convivial time in the summer sun will frequently drink far more than is good for them, and they have not discovered some special armour that will protect them from the consequences pertaining to ill health which may arise as a result of their alcohol habit. You are simply one step ahead of them and for that you should pat yourself on the back.

Rather than hissing and tutting to yourself as you make your way home from work passing what appears to be thousands of happy people getting mildly drunk and relaxing after a long day in the office, remind yourself of the likely outcome for some of those drinkers further into the night (falling over, regrettable sexual encounters, unnecessary arguments, a hangover the following morning which acts as an obstacle to good parenting and a productive day at work, remorse, and self-loathing); you on the other hand, have left such negative elements behind and are working on developing your mind and body in order to be the best that you can be, for you and for your loved ones.

Experiencing cravings for alcohol in situations such as the

ones described above is a normal part of adjusting to an alcohol-free life. There isn't (unfortunately) a magic button which can be pressed to instantaneously rewire the brain after years and years of habit-forming drinking patterns. You're stressed, you drink; you're celebrating, you drink; it's a wedding, you drink; a funeral, you drink; end of the week, you drink – you get the picture. In order to eliminate these triggers (which will be different for everyone) ample time (completely alcohol-free) must be allowed in which to nurture new and alternative habits.

I spent twenty years masking with booze any negative emotion which I felt creeping up on me like a gloomy fog crawling in from the sea. For two whole decades I never truly felt a bad feeling – I effectively froze my emotional maturity somewhere around sixteen years old, the age when I first began to depend on alcohol as something of a tranquiliser for the crap that is occasionally hurled at us during our lives.

For many people, abusing alcohol becomes normal and everyday – as unremarkable as drinking a cup of tea or eating a slice of toast. That bottle of wine (or whatever) each night fits in with life so easily that the fact it has mind-altering properties that effectively prevent the drinker from growing emotionally as a person almost passes by unnoticed. Facing challenges and learning how to cope with them in a healthy and sober way enables us to develop and become stronger with each of life's difficulties that we successfully negotiate our way through. If we fail to face up to those challenges and instead choose to drown our sorrows with alcohol, we are never moving forward mentally.

After the initial buzz of finally finding the courage and motivation to quit drinking wears off, many people (myself included) experience strong doubts regarding their decision to become alcohol-free. As discussed in earlier chapters, the rose-tinted glasses, the persuasive offers to 'just have one' from those nearest and dearest to us, and the ubiquitous nature of alcohol which finds us bombarded by images of glamorous and happy people quaffing booze all play their part in creating those niggling fears about whether we really should have given up drinking for good.

Indeed, one of the most difficult consequences of putting down the bottle for good is that you will now have to learn how to cope in a wide range of emotional situations (some good, some bad) minus the prop of booze, and it's this that could push you very close to boozy temptation once again if you aren't prepared to deal with it. Rather than wait for that tricky situation to arise – the rocky patch in your relationship, the dressing down by your boss for something that wasn't your fault, or just the rough day from start to finish that finds you tearful and dejected by late afternoon with thoughts of alcoholic beverages worming their way into your conscience yet again – take heed from the remainder of this chapter and arm yourself with some booze-beating ammo BEFORE the time comes when you'll really need it.

Physical Exercise

Always consult your GP before embarking on any exercise programme if you are not used to exercising. The following extracts are taken from the Health & Fitness page on Soberistas.com.

At school I was never interested in PE. I wrote fake letters to get out of everything, from swimming to football to hockey. Cross-country was (I am incredibly ashamed to write this now) an opportunity to smoke a load of Marlboro Reds with my mates behind a bush, around the corner from the starting point; here we would sit, stinking up our shorts and T-shirts with cigarette smoke, until the rest of the class began to pass us an hour later on their return to school. We would then tag on the end, and jog the final five minutes back to the changing rooms, fags tucked away in the elastic of our shorts.

When my eldest daughter was a toddler, I discovered running. I watched the 2001 London Marathon on the TV for the first time, and was utterly inspired by what I saw. I decided there and then to start running, pushing all the negative associations of exercise from my school days to the back of my mind.

Over the course of the following year, my sister, friend, and I built up our running abilities from zero to 12 miles. Two of us had small children, so it was a great opportunity to escape the house after a long day at home cooking, cleaning, and coping with toddler tantrums, for an hour or two of pure stress release, a good chat, and a boost of endorphins.

At the beginning, I had such a low opinion of my physical capabilities and so I couldn't believe it when I found myself regularly running five or six miles fairly easily.

My confidence grew, my appearance improved, and while I did still continue to drink and smoke (I know, I know, how stupid does that sound now?!), training for a half-marathon motivated me to keep my vices to a minimum, as the desire to improve performance was permanently in my consciousness.

The three of us all raised money for charity, and in April 2002 we completed the Sheffield Half Marathon in roughly two hours and ten minutes. For competitors who could not even run a mile a year previously, we were pleased as punch about our times.

Since then, running has been a permanent fixture in my life. I run alone at the moment, as having an eight month old baby makes it difficult to commit to a regular time – I tend to fit a run in as and when I get the chance, sometimes at 6 am, sometimes in the evenings. But whenever I go running, the following benefits are a constant, and I value this activity so much for all these reasons;

Stress Buster – I used to drink heavily to 'deal with stress' although, as we all know, alcohol actually increases stress. Running on the other hand, genuinely eradicates stress. The physical exercise, escaping the demands of small children for an hour, knowing that you don't need to worry about putting weight on … whatever the reason, running calms you down!

Weight Control – I have never been good at watching my weight long term. I can do it for a few days, omitting the cakes, ordering black Americano instead of full fat lattes, but it never lasts and eventually I cave in and get stuck into a big bun and a creamy drink to go with it. Running means that I can maintain my weight, even taking into consideration those moments of weakness.

Social Event – Though I run alone at the moment, in the

past I have always run with a partner, and will do again as soon as motherhood duties allow. If you have given up alcohol and no longer wish to go to pubs, exercising with a small group can be a fab way of meeting new friends and getting your 'fix' of social interaction.

Confidence Booster – Finding out that your body is capable of achieving goals once considered out of reach injects confidence, simple as that. In my late teens, I would have laughed if someone had told me that a few years later I would be able to run thirteen miles without stopping, and yet I can. I know that I am fit; I have the ability to commit to something and stick at it. I run in the rain and the snow and the wind and the cold – I feel fearless when I run. Running has probably been the biggest boost to my self-confidence over my lifetime; even when I drank a lot and my confidence and self-esteem were at an all-time low, running kept me from sinking completely. Now that I have removed booze from the equation, the results have been even more impressive.

Mood Enhancer – Exercise causes your body to release endorphins, and endorphins make you feel happy. Running is no exception, and I cannot recall ever going for a jog and returning home feeling emotionally worse than I did when I set off. As I have struggled intermittently with depression, I find the endorphin-boost I experience from running to be essential for my mental wellbeing – and it comes with none of the associated hangovers, bad moodsm or weight gain that alcohol used to bring.

Running is such an important part of who I am, of my life, and most definitely of my happiness and mental good health. During my last pregnancy, I missed it so much and it was with pure joy that I bought a huge, breastfeeding-sized running bra a few weeks after giving birth and began to plan my first little run in almost a year. Short of being physically unable, there's nothing that could come between me and running.

Meditation

I began meditating a few months ago in an effort to try and calm my busy mind, as it has a habit of rattling out a constant internal dialogue during each and every waking moment of my life. I had an idea that this restless mind of mine could perhaps be one of the reasons behind why I loved a glass of wine so much, as excessive alcohol has the power to switch things off mentally for a while.

Quietening the mind through imbibing alcohol to the point of slipping into an unconscious heap on the settee is not the goal that your average Buddhist monk is aiming for, and I came to this realisation around the time I knocked drinking on the head. Meditation, however, offers a mind-calming solution minus the coma, so I went along to my local Buddhist centre for a few sessions.

I surprised myself with the ease that I relaxed into such a peaceful state, especially given that I was in a room full of people I had never met all sitting with their eyes closed and feet resting atop small red cushions on the floor, but I struggled to prevent the wild thoughts (or monkey mind as often referred to by the meditating fraternity) from periodically posing a threat to the inner peace I was experiencing fleetingly but which felt just wonderful when it happened.

After a few weeks of attending the meditation class I spoke to someone who I gathered was a long time meditator, and asked her if I would ever be able to shut my monkey mind up.

What she told me was very interesting, and should be borne in mind if you have experienced the same difficulties in maintaining a true silencing of the mind.

The goal of meditation, she said, was to develop a greater awareness of the mind and how it operates, and while sometimes it is possible to quiet the raging flow of ideas and thoughts that insist on popping up out of nowhere when you are trying to visualise a blue sky and nothing else, quite often those who are meditating (even people with vast experience of the practice) do not succeed in completely closing down their thought process.

Rather than view this as a failure, the woman informed me that if I was meditating (monkey mind being awake or not) then I was meditating – with or without the restful, thought-free headspace. Becoming more in tune with your mind allows you to view it as a separate entity which will constantly produce random thoughts – some right and others wrong, some representative of you and others not – beyond your control.

This perception of the mind as almost a living thing in its own right helped me immeasurably to deal with my alcohol issues; aided by meditation, I have developed the ability to recognise my monkey mind, bad voice, devil on my shoulder, wine witch, call it what you will, and to distance myself from the thoughts which are counter-intuitive to the person I think I am and who I strive to be in the future. Rather than interacting with this negative voice, I am now able to observe it and subsequently recognise it for what it is, giving me the power to deal with it as I see fit.

This may sound slightly crazy, but I rather prefer to think of it as simply developing a well-tuned sense of self while simultaneously honing a technique which can be used whenever the need arises to ward off ideas that may thwart our plans to be happy and healthy human beings.

If you thought meditation was all about complete inner silence, think again – practicing this ancient art can prove an invaluable weapon in fighting an alcohol dependency.

Getting Creative

Shortly after giving up alcohol I noticed in myself a burgeoning desire to get creative. As a child I wrote countless stories, my bedroom filled with half-finished narratives mostly based on my beloved Enid Blyton books. I also used to bake like there was no tomorrow, rustling up ginger snaps and fancy cakes for my family each weekend, much to their delight!

As I hit my early teens and began drinking, this creative streak all but vanished leaving me with pastimes consisting solely of drinking, smoking, playing pool (in the pub, obviously), and a bit more drinking. For the next twenty years that is mainly what my spare time was filled with – drinking. Around the time I gave up alcohol I had begun to think deeply about the meaning of life, aware all of a sudden of my own mortality and dwindling amount of time left on Earth. It really crept into my conscience that drinking alcohol is surely the biggest waste of time there is, as once you are sufficiently drunk any good times that you believe you are experiencing are soon-to-be-forgotten blurred sketches of reality; they add nothing to your life or to your personal development.

In saying this, it's important to recognise that there are occasions when we do have a great time while also consuming alcohol but I firmly believe that these good times are as a result of the people we are with, the mood we are in and what we are doing. Since becoming alcohol-free I have had some fantastic nights out, laughed with people until the tears are running down my face, and danced and partied with the best of them. I have done so because I am happy, self-confident, and with people whose company I enjoy, not because I am drunk. As Lady Astor once said, "One reason I don't drink is that I want to know when I am having a good time."

As soon as alcohol has been banished from your existence, you will find that you have so much more time on your hands than you did as a drinker, a much clearer head, and a desire to do something productive. This is the time to find a creative pastime that you really enjoy and which will provide a distraction from alcohol during times of craving, when Mr Unsuitable pops back onto the scene and attempts to convince you that you should consider a reunion. On Soberistas.com members have posted blogs and articles about crochet, writing, knitting, yoga, cooking – there is a vast array of creative hobbies out there that you can now, finally, make time for. Building on your talents and increasing your ability in a specific area of interest will also have the added bonus of helping you to re-establish your self-esteem, making you feel proud of your achievements (no matter how small), and motivating you to continue with your new hobby.

In the early days of your new alcohol-free life it is likely that you'll experience strong cravings and desires to ditch your good intentions and jump back on the negative merry-go-round of drinking. However, if you are prepared for these wobbles in advance, you are much more likely to be successful in coasting straight past them and on your way to much firmer sober territory.

Exercise, meditation, and developing an interest in a creative pastime are all suggestions for the ammo you will need to build in readiness for any moments of weakness, but these are just my suggestions and may not suit you at all. The answer then is to discover and utilise whatever methods work for you – create your own bespoke arsenal and be certain to put it into action when Mr Unsuitable next comes calling!

CHAPTER EIGHT

Allowing Sobriety to Bring Out the Best in You

Much of this book so far has concentrated on how detrimental excessive drinking can be to both your mental and physical self. This chapter focuses on the positive outcomes of sobriety – what a commitment to living alcohol-free can bring to the table as far as your overall wellbeing is concerned.

There are two major aspects of your life which will be benefit greatly from your decision to stop drinking (other than the obvious benefit of your physical health), and which in turn will have positive knock-on effects on the rest of your entire existence. It is these areas that this chapter focuses on; the time you spend thinking and the time you spend doing.

Thinking Time

Absolutely anybody who has had even the smallest of dependencies on alcohol will recognise the phenomenon that is 'Internal Booze Chatter.' This incessant dialogue persistently rattling on inside your head debates all manner of alcohol-related strategies, promises, words of denial, regrets, and decisions to either stop drinking or start drinking again. It is the voice that discusses with you whether you really have a drink problem, of the definition of an alcoholic and are you really as bad as that? It is the conversation that begins with setting boundaries intended to avoid the end result of utter drunkenness and reaches its conclusion with the persuasive verbal comfort blanket which coerces you into opening that second bottle on a week night and throwing caution to the wind over the fact that you have the day from hell looming tomorrow morning.

The time we spend worrying about how much, how soon, and if at all takes up vast swathes of our head space. The problem with this is that Internal Booze Chatter occupies so much of an alcohol-dependent person's brain activity that it prevents more productive thoughts from taking place.

During the breaks you may take from drinking (as opposed to giving up for good), it is more than likely that you will spend much of each temporary respite from booze thinking about when you can next imbibe. Whenever I used to climb aboard the wagon, something I did periodically for several weeks at a time (usually following a particularly awful consequence of my last binge), I would be almost obsessively counting down the hours until I reached the end of my self-imposed booze ban – I was literally one step away from marking off the days on my bedroom wall as if I were a prisoner recording the length of time until my release.

I was a prisoner, of course, but my thinking then was topsy-turvy – I felt imprisoned by my short-term decisions to not drink as I never accepted the real mental commitment I needed to make to this lifestyle choice in order for it to work. Only by rewiring my thinking and focusing on the many positive effects that living alcohol-free would have on my life and on those closest to me, would I be able to set myself free, but all I could see was that I was missing out; let's get these few weeks out of the way in order to bring me back into the land of the living and a bloody great big drinking session to celebrate the end of my dry spell!

As soon as you flick the switch from thinking that alcohol is a substance which adds something to your life to understanding how much it actually detracts from who you really are, does the Internal Booze Chatter subside – and it does so pretty quickly. You will know when you have made that mental leap simply because the alcohol obsession you have lived with for so long will gradually decrease.

When you have made the shift from someone who is 'on the wagon' to a person who has made the fantastic and permanent decision to live free of alcohol in order to maximise their potential in life, you will free up masses of thinking time.

Here comes the exciting part – exactly what will you replace the Internal Booze Chatter with?

Since I quit drinking alcohol for good my creativity has gone through the roof. I remembered recently that a friend remarked years ago when we were halfway through a large quantity of wine one evening, that she had always regarded me as a very creative person. I scoffed, somewhat embarrassed, and threw back another massive glass of Chardonnay. 'Creative?' I asked myself at the time; 'I don't think so. All I do is drink and smoke and lurch between unsuitable relationships, as someone who was once regarded as pretty smart but whom now works as a low-grade administrator because she failed to stop boozing for long enough to strive to fulfil her ambitions. How sad.'

I lost my goals when I began to depend on alcohol for my emotional crutch, provider of all the fun in my life, and the friend who would see me through the countless lonely nights I spent watching TV alone as a depressed single parent. I had no spare thinking time in which to develop or originate any exciting thoughts or plans – my thinking was divided into two camps; a) planning/regretting/longing for alcohol and b) drinking alcohol and being drunk. Neither of these mind sets provides fertile ground for developing any creative thought processes.

My world consisted of waking up, going to work, coming home, carrying out a few chores, drinking wine, and going to bed; every day, for years. The monotony was broken intermittently by the arrival of a new boyfriend on the scene, moving house, or starting another rubbish job that I would grow to hate, but ultimately alcohol kept me in the same thinking place for about a decade.

As soon as I made the commitment to living free of alcohol I began to think so much about things other than drinking. I considered everything around me in great depth; the circle of life, what life really means, what I want from mine, where in the world I want to live, how much I want/need to travel, what is really important to me as an individual, how scarred I was from the events of my life and how much I needed to work on my state of mind, the importance of fitness and health, the centrality of family life and how it keeps me sane being around those who are closest to me, and of course, I came up with the idea of Soberistas.com.

At times I felt overwhelmed by this sudden increase in the volume of my thoughts. Certain life events such as the break-up of my marriage, which I had long-ago pushed to the far reaches of my conscience and kept submerged by topping myself up with wine every time I felt the slightest strain of emotional pain, came to the surface demanding to be dealt with. There were many occasions when my heart ached physically as I felt, for the first time in my adult life, real hurt. The coward's way out of reaching for the bottle was no longer an option and yet despite the oceans of tears I cried as I worked through all those deeply interred feelings, I realised that it was doing me good and was something that was essential if I was ever going to be truly happy and able to move forward in my life.

Of all the things that I had to process in my mind after I stopped drinking, the one that caused me the greatest sadness was the guilt I felt as I came to appreciate the extent to which I had placed alcohol above the needs of my eldest daughter (my youngest was born after I made the decision to stop drinking permanently). For months I was consumed by regrets and self-loathing as I replayed various situations in my mind's eye of my daughter on the receiving end of a mother who was either under the influence or recovering the next day from yet another binge.

I found it so hard to cope with this guilt that I eventually sought solace in a cognitive behavioural therapist and he helped me enormously. I came to realise that, while it was important to acknowledge that my past behaviour had not been exemplary, there was little point in berating myself repeatedly for the things that I had no control over and which I could not change. All I could do was learn to accept my past, throw myself into the present, and ensure I never made the same mistakes again – and that's what I did.

As the Internal Booze Chatter dies down it is likely that your thinking time will temporarily become filled with similar feelings of regret and sorrow, as you will now view your drinking history without the biased lens of an alcohol-dependent person but rather through the eyes of someone who has clarity and objectivity. It hurts – there is no getting away from that fact, but work through it and things become easier. Try and perceive this sad thinking time as a necessary stepping stone to get you to the good stuff, to the thought processes that could see you and your life completely overhauled and in a positive place where you never imagined you would go. Dealing with the guilt and regrets which have arisen as a result of a destructive relationship with alcohol is akin to weeding a long-neglected garden; it is a laborious and exhausting task but one which must be carried out prior to planting the beautiful flowers and shrubs that will transform the landscape into one of horticultural artistry.

For approximately a year following my last dalliance with alcohol, I lived in the emotional shadow of the mistakes and bad choices I'd made as a drinker. Eventually, however, I emerged (somewhat quieter and more humble, I would add) and began to live properly again. Don't make the mistake of presuming that you will feel wonderfully happy all of the time the instant that you put down the bottle; repairing the damage caused by excessive drinking takes time, patience, and emotional strength. As the weeks and months move on though, things do become noticeably easier. The thinking time that you are now allowing yourself will automatically lead on to the other great benefit of an alcohol-free life, as mentioned at the head of this chapter; doing time.

Doing Time

It is remarkable with hindsight just how much of someone's time on Earth can be frittered away through the consumption of alcohol. In my old life, every spare moment was spent either drinking or dealing with a hangover, other than the periods of temporary abstinence referred to above during which my Internal Booze Chatter went into serious overdrive rendering me unable to achieve anything worthwhile. When caught in the middle of the maelstrom of heavy drinking it is very difficult to recognise the extent to which you have allowed alcohol to run the show that is your life. Only with the benefit of sober hindsight does it become possible to grasp what a thorough time-waster booze really is.

Whether we are entertaining or socialising, on holiday, in the early stages of a new relationship, celebrating something, grieving, feeling annoyed or angry or on those occasions when we are bored, stressed, and lonely, alcohol can gradually take the lead role with us hardly realising it. Only when we put down the bottle do we finally have the blinkers removed and understand that in reality we do very little in life without the aid or prop of a glass in hand. When you have always utilised alcohol to fill the gaps in your life, removing it from the equation has the sudden and quite alarming effect of leaving you with (gasp!) empty time!

It is important to not panic and run for the hills (or in our case, the booze aisle of Tesco) when you are left with huge chunks of unfilled time that you don't know how to fill. If you allow yourself the time to think as discussed above, this will naturally lead to ideas of what to do.

Living free from the alcohol trap opens up so many possibilities and opportunities to develop as a person, and given time and a commitment to sobriety your life could take wholly unimagined turns and twists before landing you in amazing new territory that you could never have dreamt of. Doing things that are productive and worthwhile, whether alone or with friends and/or family, not only fills up all that free time but can help boost your self-esteem and confidence too.

Learning to dance, for example, or beginning a writing

course, starting a business, perhaps deciding to have another baby, writing a book (the last three are the major 'doing' events that happened in my life after I became alcohol-free), returning to study at university, re-decorating the house, sorting the garden out, learning a new language, changing careers – these are all exciting and positive examples of things that you may decide to pursue now that you aren't wasting every precious moment of life drinking, only to forget about the night's events by morning.

Not only is it important to engage in activities or interests such as those mentioned above (which are merely suggestions – whatever floats your boat and doesn't involve alcohol or any replacement substance abuse, and isn't illegal or harmful to anyone including yourself, is absolutely fine) because they keep you from the temptation of booze (this is an added bonus, especially in the early days); doing things that you enjoy and which bring you into contact with new and different people and places really does alter your perspective on life. Throwing yourself into completely fresh pastimes or ventures can have a similar result on a person's character as backpacking around the world; it can help you to 'find yourself.'

While you may have dabbled in the odd non-drinking activity here and there as an alcohol-dependent person, the booze will usually outweigh other options when, as a regular binge-drinker, you are pondering over how to spend the forthcoming weekend or evening. It is difficult to throw yourself into something fully when you are thinking about drinking wine at the other end.

As a committed sober person, entering into pastures new in the guise of alcohol-free activities has a positive impact on your state of mind because it helps you to realise that you are capable of something other than getting drunk, you can develop a skill which builds self-esteem, you can meet new people who also enjoy spending time away from an alcohol-centric environment, your horizons expand as wider opportunities present themselves to you thus providing you with new goals and dreams. These are all side-effects of activities that cannot be fully attained in a life tainted by heavy drinking. Investing time and energy into practical and time-filling interests that you enjoy will help you to grow as a person.

If not reminiscent of your own romantic history, then I'm certain that most people can recall a friend or family member who, after being with the wrong person in a relationship for years and subsequently remaining a long way from reaching her true potential, gave said chap the heave-ho once and for all, and finally emerged like a butterfly from a cocoon, spread her wings and began to live a whole new wonderful life.

Alcohol, your own Mr Unsuitable, works in exactly the same way. Its tenacious grip reaching out over every aspect of your life prevents you from fulfilling your potential; it stifles the real you. The thinking time and doing time, as mentioned above, that you would otherwise be devoting to interests and projects which have a positive impact on your personal growth and self-esteem are choked in their infancy, if they are lucky enough to get that far. A commitment to sobriety quashes the Internal Booze Dialogue that has, up until now, prevented you from thinking about anything productive or creative. The natural progression from this is that the new increase in thinking then leads to a surge in the doing.

If you feel as though your life has been going round and round in circles for years with the same old problems rearing their ugly heads time and time again, and your apparent inability to improve your circumstances appears to be set in stone as an unfortunate fact of life that will never change, STOP and THINK. Have you always drunk heavily? Do you hit the booze most evenings, only to struggle through the following day with a low-level hangover and a steely determination to make it through until wine o'clock rolls around again?

If so, and if you continue to consume the same amount of alcohol as you always have done, then you can expect the same results in life. Nothing will change if you proceed to act in the same old typical-of-you way. I cannot begin to express how vastly different my life is since I became AF – it is as though the tainted world in which I once lived was pushed through a heavy-duty wash cycle, wrung out, and left to dry in glorious sunshine, reappearing shiny and clean and injected with a completely new lease of life. I have altered from the inside out, and everything around me has changed for the better as a result (not least my close family relationships).

Despite my many erstwhile half-hearted efforts to 'go on the wagon,' nothing changed fundamentally until I flicked the booze switch in my head and made a full-on, permanent commitment to sobriety. Hanging on to a secret desire for booze behind an outward declaration of sobriety will negate any of the above occurring; the only way to bring about real change is to really change.

Arriving at the decision to commit to a life free of alcohol is, for many, much harder than actually living life soberly. Because alcohol is an addictive substance, the devil on your shoulder will work in overdrive in his efforts to keep you with him and not let you slip from the grasp of your alcohol dependency during the period in which you are considering making the break for freedom. In the event, letting go of that dependency is nothing more than telling yourself the new, exciting, and simple truth – 'I don't drink any more.'

The vicious cycle in which you have been trapped for so long instantly goes into reverse the second you make the empowered choice to live freely, minus the influence of alcohol. You will enter the virtuous circle, where your confidence and self-esteem begin to move in the opposite direction as you will now have the clarity and freedom of mind to act in YOUR best interests. Rather than perpetually behaving in ways which evoke feelings of self-loathing, embarrassment, shame, and degradation, you will enjoy the notion of waking up knowing exactly what fantastic things you got up to the night before, things that you chose to do with none of the idiocy that heavy drinking always sparked in you. Removing the shameful and regrettable incidents from life has a noticeable effect on your confidence – awoken after years spent in hibernation, that feeling of truly liking the person you are is a wonderful sensation and one that will go from strength to strength, eventually becoming a normal part of life.

Imagine spending each and every weekend completely safe in the knowledge that at no point will you fall over drunk, text or phone someone and say something that you will regret in the morning, have an argument over nothing, flirt outrageously with someone you aren't that keen on, or even have a sexual encounter with a total stranger. These things will not happen any more (unless you make an informed and compos mentis choice to do such things, because you want to) – you can relax and enjoy living life as YOU, where YOU are in charge and YOU decide how to act.

Accepting sobriety, making the commitment that is so crucial if you are ever going to fully enact change in your life, means that you no longer have to live in fear; it gives you back control. Choosing sobriety EMPOWERS you.

Being dependent upon alcohol has the effect of making someone powerless, by removing their ability to think and act freely; heavy drinkers make their choices to fit around drinking, they fail to achieve goals because they are too hungover or drunk, they fall short of making the most of themselves because they cannot stand up against booze in the fight to maximise their potential. Alcohol keeps people pushed down; it prevents those who are dependent on it from reaching out, growing and becoming who they really are. Alcohol makes people powerless and turns them into slaves to drinking.

I have never felt more able, more in control of my life, as I have done in the last couple of years since I stopped drinking alcohol. There is an incredible amount of comfort to be derived from knowing that you are mistress of your own destiny, captain of the ship in which you are sailing. I often wonder where I would be now if I had had the foresight to eliminate alcohol from my life in my younger years, but I am enormously grateful that I mustered the strength to crack my dependency at all – I now intend to make the absolute most of living as a woman empowered by finally allowing herself to be who she was born to be.

CHAPTER NINE

Long Lasting Acceptance and Positive Outcomes

There is nothing to fear from a life lived free from the alcohol trap. Anxieties over stopping drinking alcohol, which are so prevalent in the period of internal debate leading up to making the final break, are nothing but delusions and are caused by the addictive nature of the alcohol that the rational part of you wants to be rid of.

Put yourself back in the shoes of the doormat girlfriend who has been messed about for months by some halfwit who has lied, cheated, and wormed his way back into your good books on countless occasions, and because of the associated reduction of your self-esteem and confidence, you have wittingly allowed this to happen. You are fully aware in your heart of hearts that no good will ever come of the relationship but each time you receive a few 'crumbs' from this chap you are right back there, eating out of his hand.

A friend of mine explained the concept of 'crumbs' to me a few years ago and I think it applies equally to alcohol as it does to unions between people in which the power balance is very much out of kilter. The person who holds all the cards in the relationship acts in a way best described as 'slightly off' to their partner, who, picking up on the signals that they are not exactly doted on by their loved one, is eaten alive by insecurities and the occasional panic that they are walking the dating plank and will be dumped into the sea of singledom any day soon.

Meanwhile, with a growing sense of importance and assurance that they have their submissive girlfriend/boyfriend exactly where they want them, the person with the power maintains their 'treat 'em mean, keep 'em keen' mentality to great effect. Once in a while, however, the downtrodden half will decide that enough is enough and temporarily protest that this won't do and unless things change they are off. Sensing the need to give a little, the dominant one then gives just enough crumbs (maybe a little gift, or an evening during which they are particularly attentive) to convince their utterly powerless partner to hang around for a little while longer. Ever grateful for the crumbs, he or she is reassured sufficiently and snuggles up even closer.

My own association with alcohol was definitely a crumb relationship, although I couldn't see it at all when floundering amidst the sea of drunkenness and hangovers. I would regularly get to the point when enough was enough, take my empties to the glass recycling bin and throw them in with a resounding crash, full of good intentions to leave the sauce behind permanently. A few days later, however, I would inadvertently find myself in a position where I thought perhaps a couple wouldn't do any harm, and the evening would amble on nicely in a haze of boozy fun (the crumbs) leaving me positive that alcohol did indeed bring something worthwhile to my life and that no harm ever really came from having a few beers with a friend. This was an unfortunate delusion.

Ever the wolf in sheep's clothing, it would only be a matter of time until the alcohol crumb-giver would revert to type, I would get absolutely smashed and something terrible would happen. The morning would roll around and I would wake up groaning and hating myself, full of remorse and sorrow over the fact that this terrible situation had happened to me yet again, the question of 'Why me?' screaming inside my head.

The answer to 'Why me?' is simple; I chose to risk my happiness and mental stability once again in exchange for a few drinks with a friend, or maybe a couple of bottles of wine by myself in front of the TV one night. Anchoring my decision on the fluke that was the last time I'd had a few when the crumbs had been supplied, when I'd been left with a warm and happy feeling associated with drinking, I would then repeatedly make the mistake of assuming that this would now come to represent the norm whenever I imbibed.

This pin-balling between believing that alcohol was my friend and then waking up consumed with self-loathing as a result of my drunken behaviour, is what kept me alcohol-dependent for twenty years. Had I realised earlier that the odd pleasant evening spent boozing was in no way representative of my relationship with alcohol and that the darkness would gradually come to take over my entire existence each time I stepped back onto the slippery slope of drinking, I would have put a cork in it much earlier. But the crumbs kept coming, and I was sucked in time and time again.

So here is the straightforward truth – if you make a commitment to living free from alcohol, things will simplify. For those of us who are all or nothing, addictive personalities, powerless to say no to 'just one more,' attempting to seek happiness while dependent upon alcohol is absolutely equivalent to believing that remaining in a relationship with Mr Wrong who has dumped on you repeatedly but who occasionally doles out a few crumbs by way of a sorry effort to reel you back in, will bring you fulfilment and joy.

By staying in such a relationship you are willingly accepting a life spent in emotional turmoil, as your brain perpetually attempts to weigh up yes versus no, moderation versus abstinence and insanity versus calm and content.

Imagine that you are your friend and alcohol is the rotten waste-of-space lover. The friend would be begging you to open your eyes and see the truth – which is that you are a beautiful, warm, caring person who is being taken for a mug, something that everyone realises but you. Your friend can see that given just a few weeks away from this lowlife you will begin to have your self-esteem restored and the mirror will no longer reflect an image that you hate.

For reasons that are never very clear when regularly binge drinking, those who fall foul of the alcohol trap have a tough time believing that they are worth quite a bit more in life than to spend half of it in a booze-induced fog, whether when under the influence or the morning (mourning) after when hungover. What is wrong with you feeling great every day? Why shouldn't you be a high achiever who is filled with the gusto and drive required to go out there and grab your dreams with both hands? Whoever laid down the rule that says you aren't worth as much as the next person?

When the blinkers come off and the alcohol has been completely flushed out of your system you will begin to recognise that the only human being who was ever standing in your way and blocking you from becoming your amazing self, was you. It was you who picked up that bottle of wine each night, popped the cork and sloshed it into the oversized wine glass. It was you who decided to get drunk and wipe out yet another night from your life.

With alcohol eradicated from your world you may not always experience happiness but what you will have consistently is clarity. Over time it will become glaringly obvious that the only reason you felt like you were treading water for all these years was because you spent them drinking too much. The truth is frighteningly simple; cut alcohol out of your life for good and a bright dawning of reality will light up your whole existence, with the difficulties suddenly appearing easy to resolve, the challenges being - eminently more manageable, and the quiet interludes which once upon a time caused you to feel bored magically transformed into oases of peace and contentment.

A sober mind is one which is able to focus fully on the trillions of tiny miracles that we spend our daily existence surrounded by, and which when drinking heavily we fail to notice at all. I often catch my breath and experience utter awe at such everyday things as a blossom tree bursting into flower, or the rising sun spreading its light over an empty park first thing in the morning – you are not missing out on life when you stop drinking, rather you are allowing your mind and soul to absorb the incredible beauty of our world and to do so every day. Sinking your hopes and dreams in a bottle of wine draws you out of the natural way by which you were intended to live, and instead drags you back repeatedly into a darkened trap.

My life was so small when I drank, consisting of the same situations, people, and places every day of every week, a boozy Groundhog Day from which I didn't even wonder whether I might be able to escape I never knew I was caught fast in my own little alcohol prison until I eventually managed to crawl out of it and re-enter the land of the living.

Because alcohol stifles your creative mind, dulls your

senses, and turns you into something of a slave to its every whim, the real world shrinks drastically until it is nothing more than a cycle of hangovers, booze, and falseness. While you are drinking heavily you may as well forget chasing those dreams; writing a book, training for a marathon, setting up your own business, starting a class, or moving abroad – anything that takes more than a couple of hours of your time and effort is more than likely never going to happen, as just when you might approach the stage of organising everything into place the booze will come out and events will come to a drunken standstill. As a heavy and regular drinker, life becomes one big STOP sign.

Believe me when I tell you that several months down the sober line you probably won't recognise yourself – the energy that will burst forth like a fountain brought back to life after years of being blocked, could propel you on an exciting journey to places you never thought you would visit. Without Mr Unsuitable holding you back and whispering confidence-eroding messages of hatred in your ear, you will come to like the person you are again, just like you did before you started drinking in such a destructive way.

Own your sobriety and the world will become your oyster.

Making the decision to become alcohol-free has, for me, been about starting again in life. I always regarded the break away from boozing as marking the beginning of a new me, a much better version of my basic self. Adopting the mentality that committing to sobriety is the first step in an exciting adventure of self-discovery has really helped me pull through the more challenging moments, especially in the early weeks and months when I experienced (at times) a very strong desire to go and get drunk again. I felt so eager to find out what and who I would become without the constant smothering nature of alcohol holding me back that I pushed away temptation whenever it presented itself.

When you have lived for a substantial amount of time without alcohol poisoning your body and mind you will begin to notice numerous pleasing results. You will sleep better and wake up free from feeling grouchy and negative, your eyes and skin will look brighter and you will have more energy, losing the lethargy that is inextricably linked to excessive alcohol consumption. Your mood will even out and, something which for me is one of the best outcomes of sobriety, you will gradually become aware of a strong sense of clarity – and this you most likely never even noticed was missing during your drinking years. The myriad of little tasks and chores that demand attention each and every day of your life will cease to be perceived as an ever-increasing mountain of the unachievable; without booze dragging you down you'll be far better equipped to cope with those things and will simply get on with the task in hand.

Here is an important notion to wrap your head around; you cannot have your cake and eat it. The above benefits (and many more positive side-effects of living alcohol-free) can only be yours IF YOU STOP DRINKING ALCOHOL. If you were to consider for a minute that you will be able to maintain this new status quo even if you take up again with your erstwhile lover Mr Unsuitable, you would be sorely mistaken. All of these positives will be negated by the re-introduction of alcohol into your body.

This concept is encapsulated by the phrase 'Own Your Sobriety.' By taking control of your sober life, by fully acknowledging that all the good in your world has come about as a result of YOUR decision to be rid of alcohol, you are taking charge of your life and understanding the value of the lifestyle you have chosen. The two things, heavy consumption of alcohol and your positive mental and physical state, are not compatible – you cannot have both.

Once the rawness of the terrible side-effects of heavy drinking has subsided and the (imagined) fond memories of sipping wine fireside or quaffing champagne at a summer garden party have replaced the reality of waking up terrified because you can't remember the night you just had, or ashamed and anxious as a result of your inability to explain away the shocking bruises on your legs and arms that weren't there before you began to get drunk the night before, you may fool yourself into believing that this calmer life, this less moody person you have turned into, can be maintained even if you were to make peace with the devil once more.

I guarantee that this will not be the case. The key to long-term sobriety and an alcohol-free life that you truly love, rather than one in which you are simply fighting your way through each day refusing a drink out of sheer willpower and with gritted teeth, is to Own Your Sobriety. Be proud of it, celebrate all the remarkable aspects of your day-to-day life that have sprung up since you quit drinking alcohol, enjoy looking at yourself in the mirror as you admire your trimmer physique, clearer skin, and brighter eyes and take the credit for the successful and happy relationships you are now enjoying with family and friends because you are finally able to think clearly, the highly-strung, depressive, and moody characteristics you always demonstrated as a drinker having vanished without a trace.

In addition to celebrating your sobriety, a good idea is to

make friends with other ex-drinkers. Get over the belief that this is your own sordid, shameful little secret that you must hide away from the world for fear of being judged and frowned upon – there are millions of people out there who once had an unhealthy relationship with booze but who have now put their alcohol-related troubles behind them in order to enjoy a happy and healthy alcohol-free life. Find some of them – if not in 'real life' then talk to people on Soberistas.com who will understand where you are coming from and will know exactly how you feel. By sharing your thoughts on living alcohol-free, and by learning about other ex-drinkers' past experiences, you are building a cushion, a support network of like-minded people who will help you to realise that you are not alone.

Own Your Sobriety, and celebrate the many brilliant effects that living free from alcohol has on your life. Overcoming a dependence on booze is something of which you should be hugely proud, and to recognise the value of this new life you've created for yourself as a result of stopping drinking is to remind yourself constantly how much better YOU are minus alcohol. Do not take all the benefits of living free from alcohol for granted – every single one of them is a gift that you've given to yourself, and they will form the basis of a different and much-improved version of you.

I am, without a shadow of a doubt, a much nicer person as a non-drinker. As someone who was emotionally and mentally alcohol-dependent for many years, I was self-obsessed, narcissistic, and had a dangerously closed mind. I couldn't see beyond my immediate world and blamed anyone or anything for the elements of my life that were unsatisfactory. Neither did I have much of a care for the community in which I lived, and I wasn't especially compassionate – at least not if it meant actually sacrificing something for somebody else (especially my wine).

A vast alteration to my character since I became alcohol-free has been the increase in the awareness and empathy I now feel for others. As an alcohol-dependent person I was so caught up in meeting my need to drink whenever and wherever the opportunity might have presented itself that I spared little thought for much else. Being free from the obsessive thinking patterns that drinking brought about has presented me with masses of free headspace which I now very naturally devote to things and people external to me and my own needs. This, I believe, is one of the worst side-effects of heavy drinking – that a dependency on alcohol often becomes all-important, the only thing that really matters and something which ultimately pulls the drinker away from reality, and the issues and people to whom they should be giving themselves.

It seems to be a common phenomenon amongst ex-drinkers that they develop a passionate interest in helping people, or in a cause to which they can devote their time and energy. Many people upon escaping the alcohol trap find themselves filled with the urge to 'give something back' to society as the realisation dawns that they have spent most of their adult life previously thinking about booze, getting drunk and not much else.

Life became something inordinately valuable and special to me as soon as I made the adjustment to living it without alcohol, and rarely a day slips by now without me feeling grateful that I am here, fully aware and present, to enjoy it.

Breaking free from long-standing drinking habits is a gradual process during which big changes will occur in the way you perceive yourself and the world around you. Embrace these changes, learn to Own Your Sobriety, and remind yourself every day that the benefits you are now noticing to your mental and physical wellbeing are as a direct result of eliminating booze from your life. Consider sobriety as an exciting lifestyle choice which will have a major impact on the person you are and also on what you can expect to squeeze out of life in the years to come; making the choice to cut alcohol out of your life is a massive one, but a fantastic one, and viewing it as such will help you to reap all of the many rewards of sober living.

At fifteen years of age I was fairly bolshie, slightly cocky, and very optimistic about my future. Fast forward ten years and I was a slave to booze, with the worst being yet to come. Wind on a further twenty-two years after I first began to really knock back the wine with vigour, and I have recalibrated my personality and completely taken charge of my life once more.

> Making a commitment to living alcohol-free, of weathering the storms of temptation and never taking my eye off the prize of living, has enabled me to love my life once again.

For two decades I allowed a worthless, using, cheating, crumb-giving waste of space to dictate my every move – getting rid of the lowlife was the best decision I have ever made.

For everything that alcohol robbed me of, sobriety has given it back in spades.

The Sober Revolution

Part Two
by Sarah Turner

Lucy Rocca's Story

Lucy began to drink in her early teens. As someone who was drawn to other hedonistic types it never occurred to her that she, or her habit of drinking until she passed out, was anything other than normal. From the age of thirteen Lucy's idea of a night out was to drink as much as was available to her until she could drink no more – there was none of the one-off, rite of passage, embarrassing teenage drunken party incident when an out-of-character cider frenzy brings on vomiting and an early departure, never to be repeated because 'a lesson had been learnt.' No, with Lucy it was habitual heavy binge-drinking right from the word go and lessons were most certainly not being learnt along the way.

Coasting through school with little in the way of extra effort, Lucy maintained her weekend binges, and introduced cannabis into the mix too. Smoking Marlboro Reds and dressed a little like a Goth, off she trotted each weekend to get drunk and/or stoned with friends, listen to The Smiths and pretend to be grown-up and sophisticated. This continued until Lucy's early twenties, when part way through a degree course in London, she found herself falling in love, pregnant, and suddenly back in her hometown of Sheffield making plans to get married.

Despite still being young, she imagined that she had found her one true love and settled into domestic bliss, the birth of her first daughter Isobel being a wonderful and happy occasion. In those first few years of Isobel's life Lucy was the happiest she had ever been, although the drinking, once resumed following pregnancy and breast-feeding, continued in a heavy and destructive pattern.

Both her husband and friendship group were hedonists and so wild parties and weekends spent drinking in pub beer gardens provided the backdrop for Lucy's experiences of early motherhood. Although her husband was a drinker, he did not have quite the habit as Lucy did, and the frequency of which she wound up blind drunk concerned him. However, as his business took off, taking him away from his young family, Lucy found herself spending more and more time with friends (all heavy drinkers), and her consumption began to increase.

After six years together and four of those married, Lucy woke one morning to discover her husband at the foot of the bed packing his case. Unbeknownst to Lucy, he 'had had enough' and promptly left – no warning, no hints, no explanation. Lucy was left in the family home which she adored with Isobel, just four, and a young puppy. She had no job and was months away from finishing her degree with the Open University (continued from the abandoned course in London all those years ago).

The usual recriminations led to an awfully acrimonious divorce process, and at the age of twenty-seven and still recovering from the shock of losing the love of her life and the beloved marital home, becoming a single parent, and living alone for the first time in her life, Lucy fell for the charms of the bottle. The wild nights out became wild nights in, always after her daughter had fallen asleep of course, with friends popping round with bottles of wine and packets of cigarettes to help get Lucy through the early months of divorced life.

On the nights when the friends did not visit, the wine took a hammering even more than when they were there. Life became a repetitive cycle of hungover days and drunken evenings, passing out on the settee late at night in a heap of depression and heartache.

Somehow the degree was completed, and Lucy's daughter began school aged five.

For the following few years, Lucy took a low-paid part-time job in order to be around for her daughter before and after school. She lurched between relationships amidst mounting debt and a growing dependency on wine. Her reputation as the one-time party girl was slowly becoming tainted by too many incidents of terrible drunkenness, falling over in the street, arguing loudly in the middle of posh bars and restaurants, and collapsing from time to time on a virtual stranger's settee in some house, somewhere, with people she never really knew. The party had come to an end but unable as she was to admit to even herself that she had a major problem with alcohol, Lucy just carried on drinking and hoped the nightmare would end.

At some point in her early thirties, Lucy began to experience fear for the first time in her life over the amount of alcohol that she was regularly consuming. Many of her friends still drank far more than was healthy but the way in which they did so seemed more normal somehow, as if they were not engaged in the same turbulent and destructive relationship with alcohol as Lucy now felt that she was woven into.

Her life plan had been torn into tatters and hung all around her like a terrible reminder of all that she had failed to achieve in life. Despite her efforts, Lucy had never found the replacement Mr Right and had all but declared herself off the market for good as far as men went. Living in a rented apartment with just her eleven-year-old daughter, a bottle of wine had become the staple, rising to two or even three should there be an occasion which demanded the increase in volume – a celebration, a night alone when Isobel went to stay with her dad, socialising out or at home with a dinner party and wine-carrier loaded with bottles sitting in the kitchen, just waiting...

The loneliness, low self-esteem and far-reduced expectations had gradually, over the years, become the norm. Happiness and positive thinking were a part of other people's worlds – Lucy's future looked bleak and she felt with a growing sense of urgency that time was running out.

The night when it all came to a head was, strangely enough, after she had met the man who was to shake her out of her planned commitment to the single life. Filled with a sudden burst of hope that the future may not be looking quite so grim after all, Lucy tried hard to moderate her alcohol consumption, knowing all too well that this wonderful new man of hers would run for the hills if he got the slightest whiff of her certain behaviour should she continue to hit the wine as hard as she always had in the past.

The plan worked for a few weeks, with only two incidents of drunkenness occurring – one during an evening when Lucy had invited her man around for a meal, then proceeded to drink almost an entire bottle of red while cooking prior to passing out after the second bottle on the settee until morning, and the other when she gate-crashed the new chap's night out, suddenly appearing in the pub in which he was drinking with his friends like Glenn Close in Fatal Attraction, only absolutely hammered and being utterly and embarrassingly flirtatious with every man in the room.

It wasn't only these incidents which could potentially have

scared this man off, but also the dangerously low levels of self-esteem and inner confidence that Lucy now possessed. Her actions were heavily influenced by her total lack of self-worth, and as a result she trusted no-one, least of all her new partner. Convinced that he would walk out on her in exactly the same way that her ex-husband had done, Lucy was trapped by a self-fulfilling prophecy of relationship doom – keep testing, keep pushing, push him hard enough, and he'll go. Except this one didn't go – he kept on coming back, understanding her, and offering her a way out.

The message was slowly getting through, but old habits die hard, and one night when her boyfriend was out with friends and Isobel was staying at her dad's house, Lucy drank three bottles of strong wine and a litre of cider, collapsed outside her apartment on the street and woke up several hours later in hospital, her clothes sticky with cold, congealed vomit.

The doctor and nurses gave her the once over, somewhat dismissive over this thirty-five year old mother who had got herself into a state more befitting of a teenage drinker of alcopops, and sent her home.

The early hours of the following morning saw Lucy throw her clothes into the bin, crawl under a hot shower and then slide into bed, curtains closed, where she cried in the darkness for hours. Feeling disgraced and filled with an overwhelming sense of shame and loneliness, she wondered how she would ever be able to face the world again.

The only thing that dragged her back to the land of the living was her daughter, who she now recognised could have been facing life without her mother as a result of her not ending this awful dependency upon alcohol. Lucy peered years into the future, and saw herself as a haggard, drink-ravaged woman who

124

was full of bitterness and excuses for why her life had turned out so badly, and Isobel, damaged for ever by a mum who had always put booze before her only daughter.

The hospital wake-up call was enough to shake Lucy out of her self-destruct mission, for long enough to gain some clarity on the situation. Something had clicked inside her and she just knew that she would never drink again. The hospital admission had scared the desire to drink right out of her; the archetypal rock bottom had been hit.

The months slowly passed by during which Lucy felt as though she were treading water with this new existence defined by a sudden calling to sobriety. The relationship with the new man went from strength to strength, and Lucy and her daughter enjoyed a real closeness which came about as a direct result of the alcohol having been removed from the equation. But beneath the obvious improvements, Lucy was struggling to deal with the rawness of her emotions, something which she had never done since being a child owing to her reaching for the wine every time she had felt anything at all.

After discovering (happily) that she was pregnant, Lucy decided to seek counselling in order to try and put right all that alcohol had put wrong over the preceding twenty years. That, and reading masses of books about recovery from alcohol dependency, together with the investment of time and energy into creating a new way to live that did not involve alcohol in any way, helped Lucy find her feet again in life.

By the time the baby was born Lucy was well on her way to being fully recovered, emotionally and physically, from a twenty-year-long stint of heavy drinking, and was ready to be a mum again. She spent much of her year of maternity leave establishing the website Soberistas.com which offers help and support to women like her who would not necessarily have opted for the AA route to recovery but who were too ashamed and guilt-ridden to ask for help from anyone else.

Looking back on her drinking years is, for Lucy, like recalling a particularly horrible and protracted nightmare. Luckily, she eventually woke up and worked out how much better life could be without alcohol in it.

Alison's Story

I met Alison in February 2010. Aged forty-eight her alcohol consumption was, on a good day, two bottles of white wine and on a bad day the same plus vodka.

She had been on sick leave with depression from her career in radiography for five weeks. Her marriage was wrecked, her two children just embarrassed and now past trying to get her to stop. There were no options left – get help or get out, was the hopeless pleading from her husband.

Alison came from a middle-class background with supportive parents who, although sympathetic, were also completely lost in terms of how to deal with the situation. Alison told me that she knew her father drank too much but for him there had been no catastrophic outcomes. With regards to her father's alcohol consumption, her mother simply coped. There was no disassociation or dysfunction within family life.

Alison never particularly liked alcohol as a teenager and only started to drink socially when she went away to university which she did for no other reason than to simply fit in. Even then the boozing was not a regular event and having experienced a near rape when she was drunk (something which was to play a part in Alison's story further on down the line) she made a concerted effort not to party too hard.

The view of her few friends was that everything was fine; Alison was a studious young woman who was more than a little self-contained but who appeared happy enough.

Following graduation she met her husband-to-be – in banking, sharp, astute and, like her, a very articulate, well rounded person. He was eager to climb the corporate ladder and Alison was equally as keen to excel in her field. Both driven and aspirational, they forged ahead. Martin, the husband, was a very light drinker who could easily take it or leave it. However, as he climbed professionally she not only had to keep her finger on the pulse with her own work, but also had to do some serious entertaining and socialising with her husband and his colleagues. Between the ages of twenty-four and thirty she worked hard at both.

She started to notice that the odd glass of wine or a gin and tonic was becoming de rigeur for both her and Martin – when in attendance of the many 'dos' they were invited to, the champagne and red wine flowed. Alison also noticed small things had begun to slip. A perfectionist almost to the point of being a pedant, these little mistakes were making her feel increasingly uncomfortable; the alcohol consumption rose and the work ethic stalled more and more.

Discussions about children began, and they tried for a baby. It was not happening, tests showed flaws, and so IVF was offered. Alison felt a sense of real failure with this diagnosis and as a result, just like with all the other ups and downs that seemed to building up, she drank more.

A few weeks later and, realising that the barrage of tests for IVF could highlight the fact her alcohol consumption was now very definitely over the safe guidelines, she made the decision to cut right down. Despite the reduction in her intake, however, the whole preparation for motherhood sparked off an entirely new set of problems within the marriage. Martin just carried on as before – after all, he was not the one having to change. The seeds of deep resentment were slowly being sown.

Eventually the couple were graced with twin boys and joy replaced more sinister feelings for a time. However, exhaustion coupled with the conflicting emotions of euphoria that the children were healthy, together with weariness over the fact that they were oh so demanding, began to negatively impact on Alison & Martin's relationship. Things escalated to the point where he demanded and took, and owing to her depleted self-worth, she simply succumbed.

The close encounter with rape back in her university days was brought to the forefront of Alison's mind once more, as with her marriage crumbling around her eyes, any effort on Martin's part to initiate intimacy was perceived by her as mere usage. Owing to her wish to keep him from complaining about her excessive alcohol intake, Alison generally complied, although she came to perceive her husband as little short of a rapist. Her respect was utterly lost for him, and vice versa.

Alison had given up work to care for the boys, on Martin's instruction. He didn't want his children being minded by others and so as his wife's erstwhile career dwindled to nothing, he shone more and more. She felt invisible, dull, and more or less an appendage. Drinking wine as she prepared the evening meal meant she could have a head start before he came home. Often Martin would not return to the house until the meal had curled and dried in the oven, and Alison soon began to live in a separate world where she was no longer noticed, vital, or engaged in witty and interesting discussions with her husband at the end of each day.

Things were brought to a head when Martin came home earlier than expected one afternoon and found his wife at the bins trying to dump empty bottles before he had a chance to see them. Rows, recriminations, and enraged demands that Alison should never drink again, span around for weeks, but the more he attempted to curtail her consumption, the more she drank.

Alison had been a social drinker (albeit an increasingly

heavy one) until she had her children. From their first birthday onwards, the decline into dependent drinking, which was often hazardous, was rapid. She also became dependent on painkillers, Co-Codamol and the occasional use of diazepam. She was completely overwhelmed both with the drinking and

> Have you started to think about how good it will be to share your story yet? It can have a whole new ending to the live you are living now. Make the change now and start living a happy healthy life where the only thing you'll have given up will be being controlled and defined by alcohol.

where on earth her life had gone, seemingly in a very short space of time. There were no indicators or events of massive consequence to cause Alison to lose her way quite so dramatically; just a total loss of her sense of self and with that, the invisible line was crossed.

Alison came to me for help with both her drinking and the underlying causes, and has now been sober for three years. She is well, happy, back at work and thriving.

Sober, she and Martin were able to talk, although this was not without problems. However, now free from the grip of alcohol-dependency, Alison is positioned in a place where she has a clear perspective on life, and Martin's old accusations of her being unfit as a wife or mother no longer hold any truth.

Slowly, they are rebuilding their marriage. No one had seen this coming to a nice girl like Alison.

Brian & Julie's Story

Not all clients come to me directly. There is often a call from a distressed partner or parent.

Julie was a maintenance drinker. From being fourteen years old she had never been drunk as a result of consuming alcohol, rather just numb. Her husband Brian rang me when she was admitted to a 48-hour detox programme via the NHS. He had seen a feature about the Sanctuary in the local paper the previous year and wondered if I was available to offer some help. The scale of the problem was far more complex than just straightforward misuse, and I was soon to discover a secret world of seriously heavy drinking, at the centre of which was a couple deeply in love, both with each other, and alcohol.

Julie had simply never been fully sober for any of her adult life. In addition to this, Brian was also a heavy drinker and they had enabled one another's addiction throughout their long marriage. He recognised this, but had never known his wife to be any other way and for the two of them, the prospect of not drinking was a total anathema. Now in their 50s, this latest turn of events surrounding Julie's sudden detox treatment had come as a real wake-up call.

Julie had been referred by her GP to the hospital for some tests. She had always been pretty uninterested in food because she tasted little, and her stomach had been badly cramping of late with an increasing regularity. In an effort to be reasonably compos mentis, Julie avoided alcohol the night before her appointment. She had noticed that her gums had been bleeding in the last few weeks, and the acid-like indigestion she had been experiencing meant she could only sleep while propped up on pillows. She was so detached from herself now, however, that she just put these discomforts down to age, and like so many others she swept the unsavoury clues under the carpet.

Her stomach was very painful as she prepared for her visit to the hospital, so much so that Julie could barely face even a drink; she really was relieved to be on her way to have some treatment which she imagined would make everything better within a few days, leaving her free to return to the booze. She arrived on the ward at 8.30am, when she suddenly began to shake, bile rose in her throat which was followed by the vilest taste of iron, and then blood pumped out of her mouth all over the shiny floor.

The erosion of her gastrointestinal tract presented itself with darkly perfect timing. What Julie had thought had been bleeding stemming from her gums, had in fact been the result of acid from the constant flow of booze wearing her intestine walls away. She had hematemesis, a pre-cursor to so much more irreversible damage. Having blindly thought that the doctors would just fix her, the last forty-odd years of abuse had now, finally, caught up with Julie. As she told me later, although the incident in the hospital ward had been terrifying, it had also come as a relief. She was just tired of feeling nothing. At fifty-two, she could not remember the last time she laughed or cried.

The detox was imperative for her, for it was far too dangerous just to stop drinking and go cold turkey but after the detox, then what? Julie is a very private person, running her own business from home, and she and Brian had lived in a bubble of booze together for many decades. She was not prepared to share her most intimate life stories with a group of strangers in a public place, thus the options of any type of group therapy or alcohol-recovery meetings were ruled out; and so the call was made to Sarah.

Julie and Brian had never had any children, and none of their parents was still living – they only had each other. Two people, so in love and living such insular lives with alcohol binding them together, they had lived through thirty years' worth of drinking together like a couple of fish, the alcohol firmly cementing their bond. Brian was scared that with this most powerful drug of harm removed, their cocoon-like existence would implode.

The final drinking curtain was about to be dropped ...

This was one of the few times in which I have helped a couple who were both experiencing the same level and manifestation of dependency upon alcohol. Often families are involved with supporting their loved one in recovery, and frequently beset by sheer helplessness they try so desperately to understand, but rarely does a couple share so many common traits in drinking together. Many men who drink do so, at least some of the time, outside of the home with pals in the pub or with a few rounds in the bar following sports activities. Many women who drink excessively do so, at least once in a while, on a night out with friends. But Brian and Julie never drank outside of home, nor with anyone but each other; the couple enjoyed drinking together and only in the safe nest that was their home.

The only saving grace was that Brian was not as badly affected physically by the alcohol abuse as Julie was – for the time being at least.

It was almost like entering a secret world the day I first went to visit them both. Julie lived for booze, Brian, business and the garden. The thing which struck me immediately upon arrival was the sheer joy exuding from their lavender-bordered camomile lawn. There was no real order; this was not a park, just an amazing picture derived by an incredibly creative mind.

133

It was a clue to what lay beyond the front door.

Brian is a successful antiques dealer by trade, and their entire home was crammed with exquisite pieces of furniture and a vast array of *objets d'art*. It was immaculately polished, the French Ormolu mirrors glistened, and great bunches of roses picked from the garden were arranged beautifully on the tables. It was truly magical. Sitting among all this beauty were Brian and Julie, looking as if they had lost something far more precious than all which surrounded them. Both had come to realise when all was explained at the hospital, that Julie would not last into old age if the drinking wasn't addressed. Brian also understood that his drinking would have to stop too.

There was something so unique about this couple – polite, non-aggressive, placid people who had somehow never spent any time away from one another, and each supported by gallons of their drug of choice with Julie favouring gin and wine, and Brian, whisky and beer. Somehow, the toll that their drinking had begun to take so innocuously in the beginning but now so aggressively, seemed terribly unfair; they had never hurt anyone nor each other, and so deadened were their senses that it was hard to understand how their combined passions, brought to life both in the garden and in the wonderfully tasteful interiors, had lain hidden from the world for so long.

As much as I concentrated on Brian and Julie as the three of us sat talking in the drawing room, there was something out of kilter which I couldn't quite place my finger on. Brian picked up on my slightly quizzical expression, and quietly said, 'It's the clocks, I have been so pissed for so long, none of them tells the right time.' As serious as the situation was, we all burst into gales of laughter. Julie was almost crying, in part out of pain as her tummy remained so sore, but mostly they were happy tears.

The atmosphere lifted in that instant and for the first time in a very long while, Julie and Brian felt alive again. Their journey to sobriety had begun.

Brian is an archetypal Yorkshire man, sometimes melancholic but with a rapier wit. Over the years he had handled the supply of alcohol for the both of them. Buying antiques from all over Europe meant he was internet-savvy and had frequently worked out some great deals on plenty of alcohol shipped in from the Continent. As I explained to Brian that in order to keep temptation away it was best to have a completely alcohol-free house, he scratched his forehead and said 'You'd better come with me.'

Following him through the kitchen and down the stone cellar steps, I was blown away by the most fantastically organized booze bank, where there was enough alcohol in place to keep even this couple going well into 2020. I could hardly tell him to tip it down the sink; for one it would have taken days, and secondly, there was no way he was going to throw his hard-earned and valuable collection away. Yorkshire men like to turn a profit and so my suggestion of selling it all really did appeal to him. Once a dealer, always a dealer!

The sale of the cellar forced Brian and Julie to interact with people outside of work, and they'd really no idea of how curious those who lived nearby had always been with regards to the two of them and their private little world. Julie was so talented with horticulture and decided to bravely open her garden to the public as part of an annual village event which she had never previously bothered with.

Anyone who has been gripped by alcohol-dependency needs projects and interests to fill the void once the booze has been shelved, and no one filled the vacuum better than Julie. Rid of her addiction, she threw herself into gardening overdrive, and has since created one of most beautiful country spaces that I have ever seen. As she says, the precious seedlings remind her, each time she sees one determined and pushing up through the compost, that sometimes against enormous odds, it is possible to make it into the light from complete darkness. Yet, even then, still delicate and fragile, those same seedlings require such tender care in order to fulfil their potential.

There is no resentment in either of them, and because they still prefer their own company, the decision to remain dry has been less difficult. There have been no social gatherings during which temptation may rear its ugly head – just each other, with their love growing far stronger than it ever was before. Both of their libidos had been deadened by booze for many years, but now things have been sweetly restored to how they were when Julie's smile first knocked Brian for six.

> Are you ready to call time
> on wine o'clock too?

Brian still buys and sells antiques, and is now also an avid reader of vintage wine books; he really does enjoy the history of so many fine grapes, and Julie even agreed to grow a vine in the greenhouse, at her husband's encouragement. At eight months sober, all of Julie and Brian's clocks are telling perfect time.

Georgie's Story

Georgie came to see me in March 2011 aged thirty-five. She was very poorly and had been detoxed twice, both just five-day treatments, managing a few sober days following each before returning to her drug of choice, vodka.

She had never had an alcohol-free day since she was thirteen. Probably one of the most intelligent women I have ever met, her parents were academics and both drank in fits and starts. She had two siblings, one a heroin addict, the other totally unaffected by any chemicals.

Georgie had been placed in private boarding school when she was eight years old and she hated it. Since being four, all she'd ever wanted to do was dance. There was no effort to her at all, she found everything in life to be easy and she never felt challenged. At thirteen she fell in with some girls who were not as bright as she, but easily led and equally as hedonistic. They smoked and drank, enjoyed winding up the teachers, and were often suspended. The business of being a rebel became regarded as a badge of honour.

When she was fifteen, Georgie was caught dealing cannabis in school and was expelled. There was no remorse; in fact, she was delighted to be sent to a state school. She was never going to engage with authority, so carried on as she did at boarding school without the constraints of a rural setting; before long, Georgie was on fire with booze, drugs, and boys. She failed her exams and started working as a waitress. The hours suited her and her charming nature ensured she got along well with the customers. All hopes of any high-flying career dashed, the only glimmer of hope as her parents saw it was at least their daughter was still living at home where they could keep an eye on her.

This living arrangement, however, was not to last for much longer. When Georgie was seventeen, a customer asked her out. One thing led to another and before long, she moved in with him. He was as much of a party animal as she, and fell in love with Georgie's beauty, wildness, and brains. Together they dived into a debauched existence and within three years, she was a full-blown alcoholic. Drinking vodka for breakfast, the days would disappear into a fog of booze and cocaine.

Aged twenty-five, Georgie and beau were involved in a horrific car accident – she was driving and both were lucky to not be killed or to have killed anyone else, but the consequences were overtly embarrassing. Where previously the couple had mixed within a small circle of like-minded people thus their hedonistic shenanigans had been kept fairly contained, this latest consequence was splashed all over the news and on local radio.

But it did not curtail her, rather, it propelled her. There now seemed to be no need to even try to sober up and friends gradually began to drift away from what was swiftly becoming very erratic behaviour. Late-night drunken and garbled phone calls were not uncommon, and peculiar text messages were sent, bombarding friends and family with odd requests and statements. The friends who had some remaining compassion tried to get her to seek help, and Georgie dutifully visited her GP a few times but was never honest about her alcohol consumption. Despite the doctor having notes on the car accident, Georgie, when queried about it, merely implied that the out-of-hand drinking on that occasion had been a one-off. A GP has no time to argue with a drunk who is firmly in denial, and Georgie's doctor simply told her to try to cut down.

Finally the boyfriend reached his limit. Georgie was

drinking so much in the day that even contemplating a social event in the evening now seemed ridiculous. Her response to him voicing his concerns over the amount of alcohol she was imbibing was to pack a bag and leave. There was no way he was going to make her choose anything, including him, over vodka.

Back to the long-suffering parents she went. Now facing restrictions with regards to how much she could get away with drinking, the hiding of bottles and secret drinking phase began to take hold. By now, Georgie's finances were not in great shape but she managed to hold things together for sufficient time in which to top up her bank account. Unfortunately, these meagre funds were soon blown on wild nights out. Preparing one evening for what would have been yet another monumental binge, she was fixing her hair and make-up when she tripped in the bathroom, smashing her head on the side of the cast iron bath.

Kept in overnight at the hospital where her father had taken her following the fall in the bathroom, Georgie began to fit early in the morning. Immediately recognised as an alcoholic withdrawal (she was so drunk the night before that the doctors had quipped when stitching Georgie's head that they would be able to forego any anaesthesia), the consultant recommended that she be supplied with medication and be entered into a five-day detox. Without hesitation her father agreed, and was so relieved about the fact that his daughter may finally be rescued from her addiction, that he barely noticed paying the £3,500 for the treatment.

Within a month, Georgie was back on the vodka. This was to be the final straw for her parents; they could take no more. She found a flat in Harrogate and drifted between casual relationships and jobs. There was simply no control left, and a year later she ended up in an NHS facility for yet another detox. She refused rehab and the medical professionals involved were in no position to insist – their ethos is that a programme of recovery will only be successful if the patient undertaking it has a desire to be helped. Neither did Georgie consider entering into Alcoholics Anonymous, as the last thing she wanted to do was, as she put it, "... be committed to a lifetime of self-flagellation."

She made contact with me for the one and only reason that it would appease her parents. Her father had rung me months before, and I had spoken to her briefly then so I was already aware of Georgie's background. The first meeting was like talking to an automaton. She had heard so many generic questions and platitudes that she almost had a script. After half an hour I politely asked her to leave and to come back when she was ready to tell the truth.

Three weeks later she rang and asked if I would see her again. When she arrived we talked for three hours straight, during which time Georgie's inner child was released. Finally she was ready to face life in the raw. This emotionally immature woman was now ready to grow up, aged thirty-five.

Georgie had endured a very constant, extreme, and in part, exciting relationship with alcohol. Because of her veneer of confidence, even those closest to her had never imagined that there was a real need for support. There was an assumption in the early days that because of her self-assurance, the over-indulgence in alcohol was merely a phase, something that she would grow out of. Highly driven women like Georgie often have an in-built impulsiveness, meaning they perceive risk as a challenge rather than something to fear. This element of

Georgie's character further served to create the impression that she was bold, brave and certainly not in need of help.

Hindsight is a wonderful thing, but in the case of Georgie, ignoring the problem (which for a long time her nearest and dearest did) was the worst move. Under the misguided and yet understandable impression that she would grow up and then out of it, those around her largely left her to her hedonism during her teenage years and early twenties. Confrontation with a teenager who is headstrong and opinionated can be an uneasy prospect for parents who are feeling already fraught with angst. Georgina had the deepest desire to explain to me that she never once in the beginning considered that her drinking was a problem. Selective in her memories of boozing, she also chose to create excuses and reasons to justify her drinking. All of them were true, but certainly there were as many good reasons to not drink, which Georgie had clearly decided to ignore.

During therapy, the conflicting emotions were very difficult for this troubled woman to bear. On the one hand there was remorse, but on the other massive resentment aimed at, as she saw it, her innate weakness and lack of willpower. I explained to Georgie that willpower had absolutely nothing to do with her situation. She is possibly one of the most determined people I have ever met and has bags of willpower; it was just simply directed at the wrong reward.

So from late teens to her thirties, not only had she been living with a mixture of shame and rebellion but also with others telling her that she was a lost cause, damaged and beyond reason. For someone who had started out with such high expectations to be gradually stripped of all self-esteem and self-worth, the solution was just to accept that persona and drink more. Feeling so unworthy and her days characterised by the serious delusion that this was the best way to attract attention, Georgie entered into a self-fulfilling prophecy.

Her relationship with alcohol had been long and exhausting but she desperately wanted to unearth some good reasons to stop. People like Georgie who have such an attachment to alcohol often cannot imagine life without it. The thought of facing the world unshielded for this once fearless girl was in itself a colossal test of her chronically low self-worth. Fear is one of the foremost reasons for not stopping drinking, which again shows the insanity of this illness as there is little fear demonstrated while imbibing of the (frequently horrific) consequences of doing so. One of Georgie's biggest regrets was how she had inadvertently maintained the illusion of controlled use until clearly there was no control left. In addition, a complicated web of secrets and lies had sprung up as a result of this delusion, which had then become a further burden of worry.

Every perceived failure in Georgie's life was seen by her as a reason to drink, and the failures only increased with time and the level of dependence. At thirty, there was no doubt that her tolerance had plateaued and she was teetering on the edge of the downward slope. No longer able to cover her tracks or to maintain relationships, the once assured perfectionist saw the flaws build up and stare right back at her from the mirror. She had never been honest with herself over her relationship with alcohol, and similarly, Georgie was quite unable to be truthful with the men in her life. This was not helped by the fact that she'd never chosen a relationship or lover without the skewed view of alcohol.

It was imperative that Georgie learn that people-pleasing is not necessary in order to gain approval. Sobriety is largely about self-preservation and in order to achieve this, Georgie would need to be far more selective in the future in her choice of partners and friends. The majority of women are intuitive, but that intuition is lost with heavy drinking – regaining it takes time, as does learning to trust it.

Now married to the owner of a martial arts club, Georgie works alongside her husband and is currently training to become a dance teacher.

Claudia's Story

I met Claudia in 2009. No one could ever have imagined that she was anything but impressive and immaculate. There were no skeletons in her cupboard; she was married very happily to a successful businessman, had two wonderful children, a gorgeous home, and all the accessories that went with an upper middle-class lifestyle. She had a set of equally glamorous yummy mummy friends, all of whom were sociable, often volunteering in the community and who enjoyed the gym and the beauty salon. Together they followed fashion, and slavishly lavished the current trends and styles on homes and husbands.

At forty-two Claudia had it all, including a very unhealthy capacity for Pinot Grigio. She had never questioned her drinking as in her mind, units were something that other people measured and which she really had no need to. So far, there had been absolutely no reason at all to be even remotely concerned about her drinking – it was simply an enjoyable aspect of life and part of her style.

She had to admit that she'd started to feel a bit fuzzy occasionally, but her husband drove the children to school and they walked from the bus stop to home, so there were no school runs to incorporate into her day. Neither was there any neglected housework over which to feel guilty as her cleaner took care of that, so all in all, having the odd rough day was not a major problem. Often, over a couple of glasses at lunchtime with friends, Claudia would make light of the whole deal. As she told me, she and her socialite group were wealthy and protected, regularly quipping with comments such as 'Something has to kill you, it might as well be Krug.'

With such a light-hearted view of life, on the day she got her forty-third year's medical MOT back from the doctor the results of the blood tests came as more of something of an inconvenience, rather than a shock. The GP called her in regarding her liver function tests which were abnormal. Claudia was anticipating some kind of medication to sort it out, and then tally ho, everything would go on as before. She was certainly not expecting to be told that she had to stop drinking.

Not only were her blood results poor, the doctor also suspected a fatty liver, precursor to hepatitis and even worse still, the silent killer cirrhosis. So very difficult to diagnose, he arranged for a scan. By now Claudia had gone into shock. Yes, she had put on weight around her tummy but who didn't after having a couple of children? She had never dreamed that a nice bottle of wine or two could be remotely harmful – people like her could never be classed as alcoholic, could they?

There had been itching on her legs, (which is sometimes a sign of liver problems) but again this had not raised concerns as she had thought that it was perhaps a reaction to a new range of body cream she had tried. This was all happening far too fast, she just wanted to get home, and yes, have a drink to take it all in.

How could she possibly have endangered her health with expensive white wine, a drink she had always enjoyed in the same way as the rest of her social circle did? Therein lay one of Claudia's many misconceptions; in fact most of her friends only had a couple of glasses in the evening (albeit big ones) but she had gradually upped her intake to a couple of bottles. Jacob, her husband, loved his wine too, and as the children and house were both equally well-managed, he had never seen any dangers looming.

Claudia was certainly not going to tell him about her

appointment or the liver test results, and decided that she would simply wait and see what the outcome of the scan would be.

Alcoholic liver disease is a very difficult condition to diagnose. Only when symptoms have seriously progressed do the outward signs become obvious. Many people who drink too much become adept at the art of denial, and the idea of volunteering for liver function tests is far too scary to even contemplate. Often, they believe that the best course of action is to simply pretend all is well, and that a couple of weeks off the booze will make it all go away. Heavy drinkers have the act of burying their heads in the sand down to a fine art form.

Claudia was in two minds whether to even bother going for the scan, but during the week between the doctor's visit and her hospital appointment, she did decide to cut down on the wine a little. Frighteningly, she hadn't realised quite how difficult this would be and the realisation that maybe she was, after all, alcohol-dependent, made her anxiety levels rise dramatically. When the day of the scan arrived, she had reached a state of almost total panic.

All the staff were looking at her (or so she thought) with a knowing and accusatory eye; of course they were not, but alcohol-dependents generally believe that once the cat is out of the bag they will be vilified, and the defence mechanisms go into overdrive.

The results of Claudia's scan were ready the following week. Following the hospital appointment, Claudia had reverted to type and decided that there would be no more said on the matter and her liver would just mend itself. She had read something in haste about regeneration of the liver on Dr Google, and reassured, went back to the usual routines and habits.

The news when it finally came was not good; yes, she did have alcoholic liver disease; a fatty liver. This information floored her, not least because the responsibility was now all hers. Kindly, the GP suggested that she might like some help from AA or the alcohol services. Her pride was in tatters and there was simply no way she could discuss this, so Claudia thanked the doctor and told him that she would be perfectly capable of stopping drinking until everything blew over.

There had been no signs, no warnings, and no reason for her to see this coming. Drinking was fun and when she really thought about her life during the drive back home, she could not imagine what on earth she was going to replace alcohol with. It was such an easy, convenient thrill and fix; she adored the little wine cellar at home with all the special bottles that Jacob had arranged. Dinner parties were sophisticated and suave, girls' lunches gossipy and silly. Why her? She had never let the side down or been in trouble. She cried and it was true grief that drove her tears.

She told me of her subsequent searches on the internet looking for escape routes, easy fixes that would somehow cure her illness without meaning giving up her beloved wine. She tried every non-alcoholic drink she could find, wine especially, but they tasted vile to her. She disappeared from the social whirl, desperately trying to avoid questions about her reasons for not making the usual rounds. She'd had to tell Jacob the truth and he was completely taken aback, which only confirmed Claudia's thoughts that the doctor must have been acting in a way which was extremely puritanical – there had to have been some kind of mistake.

To give Claudia her due, she did not touch alcohol and spent the next two weeks miserable and bereft. She was a dry drunk.

Although she hated the expression when I spoke of it, there was no doubt it was true. She came to me still searching for a liquid answer to this, some form of controlled drinking, a way of compromising.

This is always such a difficult situation, because anyone who has once enjoyed the good times with drinking, and outwardly not experienced a downside, has no tangible reason to stop. When you have visibly been seen to have a catastrophic problem and friends have fallen away out of sheer embarrassment and shame, you can SEE what you have done. Claudia just didn't feel ill! How could such a vital organ not scream at her to stop? The unfairness of it was overwhelming.

Together we had to find a way to make her non-drinking as equally acceptable in her mind as her erstwhile habit of drinking vineyards dry had been. The main emotion she was experiencing was anger, followed closely by utter resentment. For Claudia, it was a case of 'Poor me, pour me another ...' for a while, and even though some people are very harsh about those who wallow in self-pity, this situation really had led to a complete loss of self for her. Life had simply lost all meaning now that the alcohol had been removed.

Working with the available options, we had to devise a good reason for abstinence which did not involve (for the time being at least) admission of alcohol being the cause. Fortunately, image is important to Claudia, so with great fortitude we worked out a plan of a short term health kick. She is so loved by her friends, and so very convincing with new ideas and trendsetting, that we agreed she would announce that she was going to have a few weeks off the booze for a full mind, body, and soul detox.

Not only did she change the drinking habit during these few

weeks, but she also took on the mantle of health food guru. That in itself was a distraction, and gave her leadership within her friendship group of a new phase. Jacob was not too delighted about all of this, or the fact that she had changed her meal time to the early supper with the children. It negated her habit of drinking while making his more pronounced.

But Jacob worked with me too, (their marriage was incredibly strong) and he came to realise that the new regime would be a temporary one, which was something he could live with. Preservation of his lovely wife now became of paramount importance. In the end, he was amazingly supportive and also made a real effort not to drink in front of Claudia in those early weeks. Following her healthy lifestyle-lead, he even bought a bicycle!

However, it was not all plain sailing, and there were some late-night, angst-ridden calls to me, and texts to say how cruel this all was. Often I was more than worried that Claudia would cave.

Adding to the pressure was that she also discovered some of her friends were paying more than a little lip service to this new health kick, and had not stuck to their new lifestyle plan as agreed. But eventually Claudia did face the undeniable fact that she had liver disease, and this was something her friends were not aware of.

As the weeks clicked by, this secrecy began to bother her. With clarity now restored, she realised that by not revealing the real reason for her own sobriety, her friends might be self-destructing in the same way. Secrets were not something she had ever really been comfortable with. Again, this mind set proves that not all women with a drinking problem have a life of secrets and lies, shame and guilt. Claudia had never felt remorseful, and nor had she ever hidden her drinking.

We discussed the decision to break the news of her liver disease to her friends – should she make a dramatic announcement or should she just subtly drop a couple of hints about the fact that consuming 100+ units of wine a week was perhaps not quite as acceptable as they had all thought and hope they would work the truth out for themselves? As Claudia said, not one of them had ever previously considered government guidelines or the implications of imbibing expensive wines.

She opted for the full disclosure to all of them, over a lunch awash with lemongrass and ginger cordial. The reaction was, for Claudia, quite a revelation. None were dismissive, all were concerned, caring, and although not quite sure that they were susceptible to any of the sixty medical conditions associated with harmful drinking, did take the whole story very seriously. None could grasp that their old friend wasn't yellow and bloated or that she had never been a falling-down, obnoxious, or aggressive drunk.

It took some time for Claudia's social group to review their habits, but eventually they did.

Now four years alcohol-free, Claudia is very much a non-drinker; full of joie de vivre and very grateful that she was lucky enough to be diagnosed before the irreversible consequences of late-stage liver disease. She also thanked her GP eventually; it was extremely good care, and I wish more would be as straight-talking.

Alice's Story

As a teenager and in her early twenties, Alice drank only when she was happy. Her moods were never particularly up or down, she was (and still is) a very balanced woman.

Her husband runs a large farm in the Yorkshire Dales and, from the day they married, Alice threw herself into farming life with gusto and her infectious sense of fun. Olivier had never known a woman like her. They had met at a summer party his sister had organised; Alice was his sister's new friend from university. Both were medical students and involved in a whirl of work and play, and together they were determined to live life to the limit. For Olivier it was love at first sight, and within a year he had wooed her sufficiently to sweep her away from medicine and into his world of sheep, wild countryside and, for a spot of entertainment, the village pub.

Alice was young, and so smitten with the whirlwind romance and beauty of the Yorkshire Dales that she really hadn't thought the future through. Undergoing a transformation from urban chic to tweed-with-everything, the big culture shock was quelled by a sense of adventure and true love. Looking on the bright side as ever, she aimed to keep pace as much as she could with Olivier's mother's standards (someone who could do no wrong in her husband's eyes), and she forged on.

She was twenty-three, running a home, looking after a husband and a menagerie of ducks and geese as well as coping with the mother-in-law, and her drinking was fairly typical; lots of wine, with more gin and tonic at the weekends than was good for her. However, youth was on her side, for now at least.

The situation worked for ten years. Then the cracks and the drinking began to show and have an effect. Alice could not conceive but in an attempt to maintain the happy life as it played out in her mind, she drank and laughed and in doing so, covered up enormous amounts of worry and guilt. There was no doubt that the raised eyebrows over the fact there was no sign of a baby were mainly directed at her. In 2004 she did conceive

– joy was overflowing, and the finger-pointing, imagined or not, became a thing of the past.

As soon as she realised she was pregnant, the desire for alcohol vanished, and she neither wanted it for herself nor resented anyone else drinking it. Three months into the pregnancy, in the deep midwinter, she awoke in the night with an awful searing pain. Frightened and trying desperately not to panic, she awoke Olivier and they got into the Land Rover and headed for the hospital (twenty miles away) in a raging snow storm and on ungritted country roads. The jolting and jarring added to the agonising pain and Alice knew she was losing her child.

The miscarriage still did not seem to throw her off-kilter, but what those who knew her were not aware of was that she was now beginning the slide into secret drinking. Her excuse was that she drank for sanity, and that was her mantra when I met her, still overly bubbly but with a real breakability about her. Since her tragedy, there had been no successful conception; in fact the bedroom had become a very lonely place. She didn't want Olivier to touch her owing to the huge amounts of deflected and unwarranted blame taking up her head space, not helped by her increased consumption of alcohol. In her mind she held her husband accountable for the miscarriage; he should have driven more slowly, their farm was too remote. It was crazy she knew but still she needed something or someone to blame.

Alice wanted to keep the meetings she had with me a secret. She had already been to see her GP for help and while he'd displayed sympathy and understanding, he'd put her fragile state down to the aftermath of the miscarriage. Because of her outward skilful coping, he prescribed beta blockers as she was adamant she was not depressed or drinking too much, and no further questions were raised.

I was blown away by her honesty and gentleness from the very first time we met. There was no bitterness to her. Small-framed but with the biggest heart, and such a sense of compassion and kindness, it really was a pity that she never followed through with a medical career. Her drinking had escalated to over 150 units a week, sometimes more. There was far more to it than simply losing the baby; she was lonely and completely unfulfilled. For over ten years she had tried to enjoy life as it was, and felt awful about wanting more for herself. Anyone looking in would have seen a woman who had everything.

Her deep-down sadness had always been covered up and Alice realised she would never have been satisfied with being just a wife and mother, even though in many ways that life seemed idyllic (she felt guilty about this too). Her boredom threshold was just too low; she could not bear stillness or a lack of cerebral stimulation. She could no longer face her life minus the fuzzy edges, looking in the mirror was painful and her once-fresh face was now ruddy and tired. Olivier said nothing, but Alice was her own worst critic and therefore needed no one else to point out the obvious to her.

The evenings were by far the worst, and with the rift that now existed between Olivier and her, wine presented itself as the best route to oblivion and switching her brain off completely. She had accepted her role without any question and this had been her biggest mistake. She wished that she could have expressed clearly to both her husband and his mother that she felt somehow displaced. Both had informed her that had she been honest about her dissatisfaction with her domestic role, Olivier would have understood. As is the way with so many aspects of life, the first move was too hard to make, and so procrastination became her ally along with expertise in burying her head firmly in the sand.

Once incredibly self-assured, Alice was now engulfed by her loneliness, as well as feeling something of an oddity in the village. All the women of her age had been born and bred locally and had a constant way of life that they loved. The people-pleasing characteristic, present in so many women who become dependent upon alcohol, kicked in while Alice's

153

dissatisfaction increased.

Alice embraced the conversations the two of us shared as she was completely committed to becoming whole again. Apart from loss of the baby, there was no deep unhappiness, merely frustration with herself. She was keeping up appearances while slipping into an angry and confused state. These emotions were complete anathemas to her, and the wine had been successful in subduing them with its seduction and cunning.

As time went by, however, things appeared to be moving along for Alice just a little too easily and my suspicions that all was not as it seemed were raised (you can never kid a kidder). By the third week I knew she had been drinking again, and told her so. There are sometimes subtle changes which occur in dependent drinkers, perhaps the tone of voice or a slight movement of the face, which reveal a lie. The wine had even compromised her honesty, and she was mortified by this.

She informed me that she had tried to moderate, sticking to the government guidelines of fourteen units a week, but this lasted for only three days. There was simply no way that three-quarters of a bottle of Chardonnay would ever be popped back in the fridge door. The ease and convenience of a fast-track route to oblivion was far too attractive. As has happened with many more clients, we went back to square one, and this time, having tested herself, she not only embraced the conversations but actually embarked on the work that had to be done.

Accountability to someone you trust can be a very effective method in overcoming alcohol dependency, and is far preferable to being told constantly that you are out of control. Dependent drinking can be arrested with the right mind-set, but it is always the case that deeper issues need to be addressed – the ones that caused the reliance on the bottle in the first instance.

This was another case of learning to be true to yourself, which Alice eventually managed to do. She re-sat her medical exams with absolute support from Olivier (if not so much from his mother) and is now working in general practice as a locum.

Also, the couple finally, managed to conceive again, Alice giving birth to beautiful twins. She celebrates her 40th birthday in September, and the pop of corks will be from bottles of cranberry champagne only, with no wine in sight.

Jill's Story

Binge drinking is a fairly modern expression which, for the large numbers who partake in this type of periodic and heavy alcohol consumption, involves indulging in a boozy session on at least one day of the week, more often than not a Friday, followed by regret, hair of the dog drinking on Saturday night, and tapering off on the Sunday with a few drinks over dinner. For many typical binge drinkers, Monday to Friday remain intact as alcohol-free days.

But binge drinkers take so many different forms.

Jill, aged thirty-six, came to me last year as a committed binge drinker. There was no question of her being a weekend-only ladette; she binged alone, three nights a week, a single mum who worked part time. On Saturdays and Sundays she taxied her offspring to their various sports activities and seemed to operate without any kind of problem at all. A committed runner, she also saved most of her exercise time for the weekends and on that level she was outwardly fit and healthy.

The bingeing started when Jill was a teenager at school. Her father was an alcoholic and never at home except on the weekends. He was violent, controlling, and Jill tried desperately hard to please him. His disinterest and lack of encouragement drove to her over-compensate to be the best in an effort to attract his attention and praise. Her Mum adored her and heaped on the praise but for Jill, it was her father's admiration she craved the most. He made it very clear on the rare occasions he was at home that her attention-seeking was at best tiresome and at worst, a real nuisance.

One Christmas when Jill was just fourteen she decided to get drunk – very drunk. The upshot of this was that her father laughed, feted her prowess at being able to drink like an adult, and even poured her the drink that was to send her to the lavatory to be horribly ill. She had finally hit the jackpot with him. Even while she threw her guts up, she could hear his booming; his girl was a chip off the old block. That first 'heroic' binge was to shape her drinking career.

Her father had never felt the need to be secretive about his drinking – he was a man's man, a hard worker, and because he provided for his family, completely (in his head) blameless for his excessive drinking, associated temper, and the consequences of the two things combined. Jill knew that she never wanted to be seen as anything but a nice person. Resembling her mother in so many ways (for it was she who had been instrumental in all of the development of Jill's character, other than the recent alcohol abuse), she was gentle and loving.

She left school at seventeen and found a job at a call centre. Happy to have her independence and now finding her mum's protectiveness very uncool and slightly irritating, Jill left home. Since that first binge with her father, she had supplied him with further reasons to be 'proud' of her. Possessing his strong work ethic, her strike for freedom impressed him too.

She said to me several times that she really had never worked out how on earth her parents had even contemplated marriage in the first place – until she fell into a similar trap.

The one time she committed (as she saw it) the fatal flaw of being drunk with strangers, her innate gentleness was wiped out by her body undergoing a sixty per cent rise in testosterone as the result of imbibing a mixture of mind-bending club cocktails and lager while on holiday in Spain. While there, she met the father to her first child on an evening which turned out to be a total blackout, other than her recollection of a full-on argument

157

with another girl whom she hit with an impressive right hook before being carted out of the bar they had been drinking in by a strong but equally drunk boy. Jill's next clear thought was one of sheer panic.

In a bed that was not hers, she opened one eye and took in the sight of an arm – again which did not belong to her. The inevitable had happened; the knight in shining vodka had carried her back to his room. Whether or not the sex had been consensual was anyone's guess but there were no signs of a fight. She just wanted to get away fast and so extricated herself from the bed and dressed, feeling embarrassed, humiliated, and scared. She had no idea of where she was, or who he was. There were absolutely no after-effects of the booze to deal with, only the sheer horror of what she had done.

He awoke and, although hungover, was genuinely concerned about where his companion of the previous night was going and of her mental state. So rather than hightail it, she agreed to breakfast and with more than a little awkwardness they found a café and began the conversation. Somehow there was a connection, and for the rest of the holiday they were a couple. He was very loud but at the same time protective, and whether it was the Spanish sun or the way he had drunkenly rescued her, she warmed to him, although secretly decided that after the holiday was over she would never see him again and that would be the end of that.

The sun-drenched binge drinking continued apace and was, as Jill told me, largely driven by a sense of guilt over her earlier wild and violent outburst directed at the girl in the bar, and the fact that if she reined it in now she might look more than a little strange to this new man who had really quite admired her spirit.

Goodbyes were exchanged at the airport along with the

swapping of telephone numbers. For at least fourteen days after Julie returned home to England, her Spanish escapades remained a closed chapter which had reached its conclusion as the plane had taxied along the runway headed for home.

A fortnight later she discovered she was pregnant.

Holiday trysts are a little like online dating; you really have no idea of who the people that you meet. are Apart from being truly terrified of the pregnancy, Jill's main concern was to wonder who on earth this man really was. The call was made, and to give Rob his due he dropped everything and came to see her. Fortunately he had not embellished his background and therefore there were no major shocks; he was an ordinary chap with a job in the building industry, and unlike her, he seemed very calm about the situation.

There was no question in his mind that he should take responsibility, and this only added to Jill's now heightened panic – she seemed to have gained a partner and baby without any kind of plan at all. It all moved so quickly that there was no escaping it.

To cover up her fear, she portrayed the whole thing to her colleagues, friends and family as something that was meant to be, telling them that it was an instant attraction and that she and Rob were soul mates. So convincing was the story that she almost believed it herself. Swept along with hormones and Rob's excitement, she played the part to the full and her first baby boy was born, healthy and bouncing. There had been no question throughout the pregnancy that she would drink; it had played on Jill's mind that she was in a drunken stupor at the conception, so wanted to limit any more guilt or remorse as much as she could.

Rob, however, stuck with his routine. An easy man to get

along with, he had made plenty of new friends after moving to Jill's hometown, joined a rugby club and was quite content with his weekends of beer and skittles.

Jill unfortunately got the baby blues. She dived into a deep postnatal depression, but having no real knowledge of the problem and because everyone kept telling her that she should be over the moon, she concluded that the problem must be in her head and started to numb out the awfulness of feeling like a drudge by picking up the bottle again.

Only wine, ever the social salve and not a 'proper' drink, did the trick, alleviating her dark moods for a while. But it also killed any libido (in conjunction with the exhaustion caused by new motherhood) that she had before the baby was born.

Her parents were of little help as her mother felt less than confident having the baby on her own, and her father paid no attention at all – as Jill said, until her son was old enough to drink him under the table there wasn't a hope of bonding.

The rows began about sex, or rather the lack of it. The excuses started to wear thin, after all their two biggest attractions had been that and booze. Now the booze remained but the love, which had never really been there for Jill, had disappeared into the ether.

They separated, and yet more recriminations surfaced. Never correctly diagnosed with PND, the blame game began in earnest. Always reluctant to talk about how she felt, Jill became very defensive and in doing so, isolated. When she drank, her attitude was that it was her and her son against the world, and when she didn't then it was the world that was against them. Occasionally the two collided and the subsequent confusion could only ever be washed away with a few bottles of Shiraz.

Those that ensued became Jill's 'Sex and the City' years,

with a little Bridget Jones thrown in for good measure. The divorce from Rob was quick and amicable and their little boy spent time with them both. While he was with Jill, she rose to all the challenges of single parenthood and ensured her son was safe and loved, and things were fine. When he went to his father, it was Jill's default to hit the ethanol, and so good was her control that she would only imbibe on those child-free days and nights, although she did so with real gusto. Jill was on a mission, comparing and competing with her peers, and secretly searching for her Mr Big. For Jill, the binge drinking came as a relief after the stresses of her marriage and the ensuing divorce, and appeared to her for the most part to be unproblematic.

Mr Big did eventually come along in the shape of Richard, whom Jill fell for hook, line and sinker. He was very charming, very controlling, and a heavy drinker. He schmoozed her, she was totally smitten, and at thirty, as they were both becoming a little bored of being singletons, they married.

His demeanour changed almost as soon as the ring went on her finger. They both got drunk on the honeymoon, and he hit her. Hard. He carried on hitting her, his punch bag now this lovely vulnerable woman. History was repeating itself, something Jill recognised, the only difference being that she found solace in wine whereas her mother had never had an escape route. Only drinking when Richard was away and her son at home but in bed, she allowed herself to disappear for a few hours of nothingness and numbness.

He didn't beat her when she fell pregnant, just abused her emotionally. Jill continued to drink throughout the nine months, although not with the same intensity as before. She desperately wanted to hang on to her only place of sanctum which had, by now, become of great value to her. Her baby girl was premature, the postnatal blues returned with a vengeance and to make matters worse, Jill now found herself belittled and also blamed for not giving Richard a son. The physical abuse resumed, with even greater force than before.

And so Jill made her escape. Without a word to anyone, she left her son with Rob, something which had been pre-arranged as a regular custody day, and drove to the only safe place she could think of to go, her parents' house. He father was ill but now it was her mother's attention she needed, badly.

Richard wanted her out of his life completely and with great alacrity settled their divorce, stating no desire to maintain contact with their daughter. A new life began.

Jill put the brakes on her drinking for a short while, trying to prove that she was in no way addicted – how could she be? For a couple of weeks, sometimes longer, she wouldn't touch a drop but there was always the thought in her mind of the ultimate and alluring sanctuary of alcohol, and its power to enable her to climb above the pain of emotion.

With the courage that so many women who go through domestic violence frequently demonstrate, she used her last resolve to begin again; she was raw, but determined to forge a new life for herself and her two children, minus the complications of any man.

With her self-esteem and confidence at an all-time low, Jill felt no guilt or shame, or indeed anything at all. Emotionally she had died. The violent battering and the chemical assistance which had only served to prolong the agony now ensured Jill operated merely on automatic pilot and no more.

She came to me after being convicted of drink-driving, something which had occurred the morning after the night before. The control she thought she had so cleverly executed all along had finally come unstuck. The delusion that her binge-drinking nights which ended before 11pm would leave her in the clear the following morning was shattered. The maladaptive behaviour, which to Jill had become so normal and acceptable, could be no more.

Jill was not an alcoholic or physically dependent on booze – she was self-medicating to the point of hazardous drinking. How can a mother ever explain to a generic alcohol-treatment service the gut-wrenching history of a relationship that was devastating both to her and her children, and admit that yes, history had repeated itself? So private, so intimate, and so very difficult to explain, the fact of the matter was that alcohol was not the most devastating piece of this story – rather it was the excruciating and hidden pain that stemmed from a father's refusal to love his daughter as she deserved. Sadly, that damage will take many years to resolve but Jill is now slowly finding her feet without any mind-altering chemical affecting her ability to make clear and considered decisions in life.

> Are you ready to be a pioneer of the 'new normal?' Living a happy, healthy life that is alcohol free?
> Come and join
> The Sober Revolution!

Rob and Jill made a fresh start, and he no longer drinks on a regular basis.

Ruth's Story

Ruth had always been lucky. She enjoyed a happy and financially comfortable upbringing, was perennially easy-going with a bubbly personality, and lived a life that was full of hope and optimism. An only child, she was adored by two wonderful parents who backed her fully in all she aspired to. From an early age she had wanted to fly high and everything she did was with great gusto and determination – including, alas, her drinking career.

She entered the world of banking aged twenty-two, a little in awe of some of her male colleagues but certainly never feeling like the underdog. It soon became apparent that the drinking culture within the finance industry was taken very seriously, and schmoozing was all part and parcel of the work hard, play hard, ethic.

Fiercely independent with no desire for marriage or children, Ruth totally zoned in on her work and rose very rapidly through the ranks. She had a lovely home, great job, close, funny friends, wonderful holidays, and passing dalliances with men, many of whom were very forlorn when she gave them their marching orders. Never had there been a truer expression, Ruth indeed 'had it all.' That is, until she almost lost the lot to alcohol.

Throughout her twenties handling the drink was a walk in the park. It was very rare she felt off-colour as a result of alcohol and Ruth got on with sinking a bottle of Shiraz at home most evenings or enjoying a few glasses out and about, and as she did so, gave little thought to keeping her eye on the number of units she was consuming. She was praised for her capacity to drink with only a few minor mishaps ever occurring; she had the odd giggly moment with girlfriends about memory lapses, but nothing more sinister came about as a result of her regular imbibing. Many of her older colleagues often found themselves in embarrassing situations because of their own excessive boozing which Ruth felt a little uncomfortable about; she found their behaviour to be somewhat excruciating and thought they should know better at their age. Pah, she would never end up like them!

I have seen a real shift in so many women over the age of thirty who drink heavily, witnessing their initially high tolerance levels beginning to decrease almost as soon as they leave their twenties behind. This shift occurs gradually at first but then with such rapid descent that the sudden shock of discovering they are, in reality, dependent on booze truly frightens them – either into getting their drinking under control, or drinking even more as the denial takes a grip.

Ruth neither denied nor hid anything – she just drank because that was the culture in which she was immersed and she rather enjoyed it. After a particularly heavy session one weekend which finished around 8pm on Sunday, she got an early night in readiness for the following morning's drive from Leeds to a meeting she was to attend in Oxford. The next day in the bright April sunshine, she turned into the main road from her cul-de-sac and down to the traffic lights at the bottom of the hill.

The lights were red, she braked gently, and without any warning there was a bang from behind; she had been rear-ended. Unhurt but seriously angry, she got out of the car to confront the idiot who had smashed into her. He was an elderly gentleman who was deeply apologetic and took full responsibility. Ruth just wanted to leave as there was not much damage to her car, and so quickly asked for details as the queue of traffic behind them was now long and commuters were becoming irate. All of a sudden, a police car drew alongside and asked if both of them were OK. Ruth was slightly flushed and feeling a bit dizzy.

The policeman, who was standing close to Ruth and facing her, asked her to step around to the side of the patrol car where he pulled out a breathalyzer. She had no issues at all about taking it, sufficiently deluded to believe that she'd had plenty of time to become alcohol-free; it was, after all, 6.30am. What she didn't know was that just one bottle of wine can take eleven hours to leave the system. She blew, and was two and half times the legal limit.

Shock and total disbelief took over as Ruth was arrested and charged with drunk-driving. She had travelled just four hundred metres from her front door. It took her some time to collect her thoughts and protest, but it was all to no avail; this totally self-assured woman of thirty-six was now going to have to face the consequences of a lifestyle-damaging turn of events. Charge sheet in hand and shaking profusely, she arrived home and sunk into the sofa clutching a very large glass of wine (the natural reflex still completely in place). Parents were telephoned and, appalled, they alerted the family solicitor. Ruth then considered her options with regards to her work.

The next move was to call the bank. Her self-assurance, occasionally perceived by some as verging on arrogance, had almost always been admired but was now about to be considered wholly inappropriate. As Ruth simply explained very truthfully what had transpired, she was expecting sympathy and exclamations of what terrible luck she'd had. Instead, the receptionist was more than a little frosty, and within hours Ruth discovered to her horror that she had been suspended on full pay, pending the outcome of the charge.

Ruth was well-known throughout the company for which she worked and soon the judgements were in full flow; within hours, the news was all over the office. Her emails and messages took on an incredibly invasive tone while all that swirled around Ruth's head was the question of 'What the hell just happened?'

For the first time ever she felt true shame and complete loss of self. It was almost as if the person who had committed the drink-driving offence had nothing to do with her, was a separate entity altogether. Ruth felt as though she was looking in at the whole mess from the outside.

The days and weeks that followed were largely drink-fuelled, the drunkenness interspersed with occasional moments of clarity during which she tried to make contact with old friends at the office, all of whom acted towards her in a manner which was distant and cold. Not once did Ruth believe that any of this had been her fault but that of unreliable police equipment, a stupid old man, and a unique (for her) stroke of bad luck.

Sinking into a deep depression, life tearing into further tatters with each passing day and her parents out of their minds with worry, Ruth was in court within four weeks and banned from driving for eighteen months. That nail in the coffin sent her into overdrive, and armed with vodka and token orange juice so began the process of self-destruction, quickened by the extra strength of alcohol by volume. The demented spiral was, she said, of near lunatic proportions. Ruth made late night calls, sent enraged emails at 3am to people who had really never done her any harm but who she decided needed to share some of her pain and torture, and made wild online purchases. Of these, the purchasing of the most bizarre products became a mere idle pastime, with Ruth buying flying lessons, vast quantities of shoes, and a weekend away for her parents at a ski resort in Scotland (neither had ever learned to ski).

Recommended to see me by her local GP after she angrily demanded anti-anxiety pills at the surgery, Jill's defences were now firmly in place. As far as she was concerned, the whole business was a bizarre dream which would somehow disappear all by itself. She was full of self-pity and completely convinced that none of what had happened was due to alcohol misuse at all, but just a stroke of extremely bad luck.

There are rare occasions when it is appropriate to knock someone down to build them back up, no matter what catastrophic consequences have been wreaked. Sometimes, taking responsibility for disastrous events which are absolutely your own fault is a bitter pill to swallow. Even the reality of a DUI had not rung alarm bells for Ruth with regards to her alcohol addiction, and she continued to maintain that she had simply been in the wrong place at the wrong time. It was becoming evident that the tough love approach was not going to work with Ruth.

Stigma and judgement can drive people like Ruth into deep denial. It was imperative that she understood the fact that, although prior to the offence she was abusing alcohol, she had not then been drinking alcoholically – harmfully yes and occasionally hazardously, but not as she had come to since the car accident. The alcoholism had crept up with great stealth and within a very short time indeed. She was now riding the elevator that went only one direction; down.

Far too many people are classified as alcoholic when they

really are not, and it can be extremely damaging to herd everyone who abuses alcohol under that same heading. Just when the invisible line is crossed no one can predict – it can be a one-off or a series of events that pushes us over the edge. For Ruth to accept that she was now alcoholic took enormous honesty and patience, for how do you admit when you are a control freak that you are completely out of control? For Ruth, it was tortuous to acknowledge that her golden future which had been lain mapped out before her was suddenly shaken to its core by this, her bête noir.

She was so far away from being a secret drinker a few months ago that she could not wrap her head around the transformation which had occurred from successful career woman to this very poorly wreck, who only ever left the house for booze and shunned all callers, including her ever-supportive parents because 'they just didn't understand'. So engrossed in overthinking the rest of her life while fuelled by the ethanol, the ultimate option of suicide was looking increasingly attractive.

The weight had piled on, Ruth's face was bloated and her eyes were filled with sadness, and yet she still continued to champion the cure-all in a bottle. I felt strongly that the only way to stop the self-destruction was to avoid patronizing her or instructing her to not drink, but to somehow restore the choice in Ruth's mind in order to build a sense of control again. We had to work for literally ten minutes at a time in the first few days; there was true despair and grief, but when she cried to me saying that the decision to live or die had now become difficult, I knew that she would get better. The illusion of alcohol being a solution was evaporating.

The old adage of it being darkest before the dawn rang true for Ruth, and within a week, she was taking small steps towards her recovery. She ceased to make the drink-fuelled phone calls and send the hate-filled emails, although suffered a major withdrawal in doing so. In some warped way, her efforts to try and justify the drink-driving to colleagues and friends had, in reality, done far more damage than the driving conviction itself. Lies told to justify actions never works, but Ruth had come to lean on this method as a way of venting her anger and frustration, and giving it up proved more difficult for her than she had previously imagined.

After three days sober she returned to see her GP and succumbed to liver function tests. Of course they came back abnormal – there was evidence that her liver was not in good shape but, she was informed, it would repair itself as long as Ruth remained alcohol-free. I had noticed there was a manic side to Ruth coupled with signs of Obsessive Compulsive Disorder (OCD), and after my six weeks with her being clear of alcohol, she was diagnosed as being low spectrum bi-polar disorder. That old pal in a bottle really can mask a plethora of other mental health issues, which can (when they are visible and not disguised by excessive alcohol consumption), with the skill of good practitioners, be managed so successfully nowadays.

Ruth held on to her job, although was monitored closely. She had to eat a lot of humble pie but that was a small price to pay after what could have been such an incredibly tragic downfall – not just for her, but for her parents too. The frightening truth was that Ruth could have easily killed a complete stranger while believing she was fully capable of being in charge of a lethal weapon, her car.

Ruth said to me 'It cannot be stressed enough how much this alleged pleasure can cause so much heartache to so many. So devious in its attraction that even the most selfless among us, and I wasn't one of them, are convinced that we are only hurting ourselves, and we would rather be fired up with wine than face life and all that it dishes out with honesty and responsibility. Really, what is the worst outcome of that way of life? I do get scared, but only of drinking again. In many ways I am grateful too because I never really understood what an unthinking, self-centred person I had become, and that apart from work, I had nothing but drink. That was a really big wake-up call.'

Ruth is now six years completely sober, and married with twin boys.

Sarah Turner's Story

Sarah started drinking with conviction when she was sixteen. She never worried that there would be any downsides to this decision as both her parents were practised drinkers and had a great social life, and although she knew that losing her twin brother at two in tragic circumstances had had some kind of an effect on her Mother, she wasn't quite sure what that might be.

Daddy looked after everything and Mummy had people who looked after her, the home, and very often Sarah too. That set of circumstances did change when her father died when she was just thirteen, but no one really communicated the reason for his death, or what a difference it would make to her mother's already fragile mental state. Sarah lived in her own world of books, ponies, and imagination. Attention at all times it seemed was concentrated on her elder brother, as well as the one her mother had lost.

She got very drunk on a ski trip in Austria at sixteen, and the drinking seemed to make everything funnier and more light-hearted. Having been a quiet child, all of a sudden Sarah found her voice, her booze head. She quickly warmed to the idea of being the centre of attention, an unexpected but happy side-effect, and her destiny was set; no more boring books or studying hard, it was party time.

She was never alone again. Having discovered that boys and booze were happy to look after her, she let them. In the latter part of her teenage years drinking was not a massive part of her life but it did seem to propel her into being far more uninhibited and full of fun.

Her mother was now firmly in the grip of prescription drugs and spirits but her only daughter had never known her without them, so simply continued trying to please her. Sarah was perpetually driven by a desperate need to keep those around her happy, feeling as though she was letting the side down if she didn't.

She met her first husband via her mother and was pushed into a marriage that would never have worked – he was much older, far more sensible than she, and her mother's choice. He rarely drank and expected his nineteen year old feckless bride to kowtow; it was never going to happen, and after realising the awful mistake she had made Sarah left him for another older man. This one was of a completely different mind-set, having both feet firmly planted in Party Central.

Sarah's drinking had not been especially ramped up until becoming involved with this new man but suddenly, before she knew what had hit her, her drinking nirvana arrived. She had a great job which she didn't really need financially, and her lifestyle was typical of the late 70s and early 80s era of liberation, excess, fun, and hedonism. Living in a city for the first time and frequenting all night parties on a regular basis, she had never experienced such a choice of drinking venues. Gone was the village pub, now there were achingly cool clubs and trendy bars springing up everywhere and cliques of people who were as hell bent on pleasure-seeking as she was.

With all this excitement plus plenty of foreign holidays to the most desirable locations, Sarah felt she had been let loose in her very own sweet shop. Spurred on by her boyfriend, they became a glittering pair on the Leeds social scene, and with all around her buzzing with laughter and life, there was nothing standing in her way. Sarah's boyfriend was funny, outrageously flamboyant, and (in actual fact) slightly mad.

His mother, an aged hippie and artist whom Sarah adored as

173

she was the polar opposite of her own, very upper middle-class mother, had a farm in Ibiza. Summers were spent there getting hammered and tanned, dancing and drinking all night at the famous clubs, wearing underwear as party wear and sleeping all day on the beach. There were no consequences except peace and love.

Things were about to change. Shortly after her twenty-fifth birthday Sarah was driving to her mother's house on yet another pleasing mission, armed with a bottle of Bell's as had been requested. Hungover, she lost control of her Mini which then skidded, and in slow motion the car and she somersaulted across the country road and through a post and rail fence. The next thing she remembered was being dragged out of the wreck (reeking of Scotch) by a heavy-set chap who ran with her in his arms away from the vehicle, which then promptly burst into flames.

Sarah had always said that angels must be watching over her.

Her rescuer turned out to be the local policeman who had been off-duty at the time of the crash, and knowing Sarah and her family (as well as their collective drinking habits), he drove her to her mother's house where they all expressed amazement over the fact she had come out of the accident with merely a jauntily angled collar bone and nothing more serious. As it soon became apparent that neither Sarah nor her mother was in a fit state to drive to the hospital, the policeman took Sarah himself where she was informed that her collar bone was broken.

That accident really did not have the impact it should have done. In fact, at the first opportunity she was nursing her aches and pains with a large gin and tonic, topping up the strong painkillers that had been administered by the doctors.

The high life went on until it became clear that no marriage or family was on the cards for Sarah as long as she remained with her present beau. Now thirty and longing for her own family, she gave him the heave-ho and soon after met and fell in love with her husband, now of twenty-seven years, Michael. He was capable of hard work and play too but did also want to settle down with her – before long they had planned their future, bought their for- ever home, and Sarah discovered she was pregnant.

Yet another dream came true when the newly-weds moved into an idyllic old farmhouse, where they inhabited a world filled with interiors decked out in 1980s staple Laura Ashley, dinner parties, Sarah's beloved Aga, and a little smallholding; horses and dogs made everything picture perfect. Wine now was the drink of choice, and there was lots of it. White and dry, it was never considered 'proper' drinking as everyone around them imbibed in similar quantities and no one seemed to outwardly suffer.

Sarah didn't drink throughout her pregnancy, other than the odd Guinness as recommended by the midwife, and soon a bouncing and beautiful baby boy was born. The champagne corks were popped, and the drinking dance began once again.

Michael was a heavy drinker too, and between the two of them the alcohol consumption was gradually escalating. Michael was also now under huge financial pressure, although he was, for the time being at least, successfully hiding this impending disaster from his wife.

Sarah had gone through a big shift in hormones since giving birth and at thirty-four her tolerance of alcohol was slipping rapidly. There really was no warning prior to her falling over the invisible line of heavy drinking into the grip of alcoholism;

175

it just happened.

The late 1980s/early 1990s recession hit, the economy crashed, and with it went their property portfolio. The security for their numerous bank loans was called in and the couple waved goodbye to their beloved family home. This was the catalyst that pushed Sarah to dive into oblivion. Her son was cared for and never in harm's way and Michael refused to take any of his normally frequent business trips. Through the worst of times Sarah tried to seek help, initially from the family GP. He was sympathetic but had only two suggestions to offer; cut down, or go to AA. Neither was going to work for Sarah – moderation was impossible for her and while she did look into Alcoholics Anonymous (admittedly very briefly), she discovered that it would take her a good forty minutes to drive to the nearest meeting but more importantly, she just couldn't see how she would ever be able to commit to such a rule-based, quasi-religious group.

Friends seemed to have fallen by the wayside long ago – her alcoholism had become so isolating that there was no one left to talk to. The few who had not vanished into the ether were all heavy drinkers too, and looking to them for support in helping her to stop would fly in the face of all that they'd shared and had in common.

In the meantime, Michael had located an ex-Skid Row bum who was now running a rehab centre on a shoestring in West Yorkshire. Although Sarah was terrified of having to leave her baby and the isolated bubble in which she had lived for so long, her choices were few and so she ended up being taken like a lamb to the slaughter (or so she perceived it) on this latest effort to find help.

There was something very powerful about this once down-

and-out man, and he inspired Sarah greatly. It had nothing to do with official expertise as he possessed no formal qualifications; there was simply a basic good inside of him together with an innate understanding of Sarah's addiction, and the penny finally dropped. She left sober and remained so for the following ten years.

Michael during that time suffered four heart attacks and underwent quadruple by-pass surgery. They downsized dramatically and took hold of life by the scruff of its neck, both gaining strength from one another. They had little in the way of possessions but material belongings had, by then, become ultimately trivial for Sarah and Michael. The only things they now prized were their family life and collective health.

Unfortunately, the drinking story was not over yet. No one ever knows why some people decide to pick up a drink again; excuses and reasons are always available if required and Sarah simply decided that the time was right, and so she did it – one glass of really good Merlot, where was the harm in that? Within a week, however, she was sneaking out for a bottle of Smirnoff. The hazardous drinking had begun again at full throttle and every single thing she had learned about her old addiction flew out of the window as if it had never happened. No one was more shocked than her, or so cataclysmically ashamed.

The fear of stopping was powerful, but Sarah set about getting on with becoming sober again and this time decided she would do it her own way. All of her life she had succumbed to being told what was best for her, and now felt it was imperative that she take back the control. Learning everything she could about this devious illness was her only remaining option – she was familiar with all the tricks and tips, and she knew the alcohol-counselling script by heart; now she needed the science and logic to provide her with the practical edge that had always been missing.

So she studied, hard, and eventually qualified as a cognitive behavioural therapist and addictions counsellor. Sarah has beaten her addiction and the breast cancer that hit a few years later. In her words, "The cancer was a breeze to beat in comparison to, not just alcoholism, but the fight against both it and all the taboo that still surrounds it."

Part Three
by Sarah Turner and Lucy Rocca

Last Orders

Between 2003 and 2012 the number of cases of breast cancer attributable to alcohol consumption in the UK rose from 9,100 to 13,700, approximately a 50% increase in just under a decade. Hospital admissions for alcoholic liver disease for the same period jumped from 25,700 to 49,500. [1]

Clearly the message that excessive drinking is harmful is not getting through, at least not sufficiently to ensure people cut down on the amount of alcohol they consume. Could it be that statistics alone, however frightening and conclusive, will never be powerful enough to combat the grip that alcohol holds over so many?

We embarked on writing this book together with a shared and firm belief that a one-size-fits-all approach to beating alcohol dependency is not effective. People drink for all sorts of reasons and their levels of dependency alter too – what may work in beating an alcohol addiction for one person, a social binge drinker for instance who frequently blacks out and suffers from depression and anxiety issues, would be unlikely to be effective for a person who drinks alone, topping up throughout each and every day, or one who consumes extreme amounts of a favourite tipple after the workday is done and the kids are in bed. People who drink heavily do so for a multitude of reasons,

---

[1] Figures based on: Hospital Episode Statistics, Health and Social Care Information Centre

using the alcohol to disguise deeply buried issues that have been interred for years; it is these personal problems which we need to address if we are to be successful in tackling alcohol dependency.

In writing this book we were also driven by a desire to normalise sobriety in the same way that our culture has normalised heavy drinking, and to make being a non-drinker an attractive lifestyle choice rather than it being perceived, as it is by many, to be a hardship or a form of martyrdom combined with a fear of missing out and being boring. We were determined to show that not all women who drink heavily should be grouped within the same category; there are big differences between those of us who misuse alcohol, and there is a wide variety of reasons for engaging in a destructive relationship with this freely available and completely socially acceptable drug.

Over the last few decades it has become fashionable to be a wine drinker, all of us having been bombarded by clever marketing alluding to the fact that wine is not only healthier than spirits, but that it makes us more sophisticated, attractive, cultured, and relaxed. Tea time has gradually morphed into wine time.

However, if our drinking careers started in earnest back in our teens or early twenties, then each emotional event that occurred during the years that followed was most likely dealt with by swiftly polishing off a glass or two of chilled fizz or room-temperature red, and common sense surely tells us that engaging in such a habit will result in emotional immaturity. Our feelings are dumbed down, numbed, or blacked out completely every time we consume too much booze. Each relationship that we embarked on probably began with a

180

romantic drink, each dare with Dutch courage, in every difficult conversation we anesthetised ourselves, and all the heartbreak we were struck down with was drowned out, washed away, and never truly lived through. All the weddings, funerals, and celebrations we attended were fuelled by ethanol, all the life-changing decisions we made warped by a bottle or two of Pinot.

Alcohol stunts our personal growth and after years of drinking heavily our default emotional state will be at best slightly immature, and at worst, defined by an utter inability to cope with life's rich tapestry of ups and downs without our crutch, this ubiquitous drug by our side. We are not questioned for spending our money on it, we cannot be arrested for scoring it and who could possibly blame us for drinking it? There are always a myriad of worthy excuses to choose from whenever we are faced with a need to justify our alcohol habit.

Drinking was, for both of us (as has been the case for most of my clients), a symptom with a multitude of causes. We never set out to be drunks but simply drank to be able to fit in, enjoy a buzz, and lose our inhibitions, and to numb out an awful lot of emotional pain. Ostensibly, living with fuzzy edges was a good way to escape the reality of life in the raw. There are so many layers to this widespread substance abuse that no apparently definitive diagnosis of 'alcoholism' can ever do it justice.

Promoting sobriety as a lifestyle choice by telling people that, without alcohol, they will instantly acquire extra sparkle, feel brighter and have more energy, falls far short of the mark. Unless a drinker undergoes a shift in her perception of alcohol, the danger exists that she will simply settle into life as a (usually miserable) 'dry drunk,' resentful and bitter that she cannot be 'normal' and determined to regret for ever not only starting to drink heavily, but even more so that she had to stop.

181

This is not a solution but torture, and we strongly desire to reconfigure people's perception of sobriety, making it an optimistic and healthy route to inner peace and happiness, rather than the lifetime of self-flagellation for events past which, sadly for some, living without alcohol becomes.

For the most part, the women who seek help from us are emotionally addicted to alcohol, with very few being physically dependent. This book, we hope, will help women to recognise before the wheels fall off completely that there is light at the end of the wine cellar and that with the right mind-set, adopting a sober lifestyle is a great option to choose. Intervention is infinitely better than any potential cure.

Below are just a few of the different 'types' of drinkers. This is not a clinical view, but one drawn from real life experience and from working with women who have been brave and honest enough to discuss their drinking histories so candidly.

BINGE DRINKER

Over the last twenty years, the binge drinker has featured in many a newspaper column, and especially so for young women. If these women survive the dangerous situations that they often land up in as a result of a night out boozing, then alcoholic liver disease may catch up with them during their thirties or forties instead, the increase in this condition amongst younger females borne out in the latest statistics.[2]

We wanted equality, and in many areas of our lives there has been an increased parity between men and women, but the fact

---

[2] JECH Online First, published on July 18, 2013 as 10.1136/jech-2013-202574

remains that women just cannot drink on an equal footing with men. Of particular importance is the fact that women who regularly drink three glasses of wine a night increase their risk of developing breast cancer by a whopping 50%. In addition to the above-mentioned dangers, binge drinking often has other, more immediate, negative repercussions too; relationships break down over a drunken row and jobs are lost due to regular absenteeism. Binge drinkers will frequently climb aboard 'the wagon' for the odd week of detox and flushing out their systems with plenty of water, before embarking on a massive alcoholic blow-out when they reach the end of their self-imposed Spartan living to celebrate their return to Vino Land.

HARMFUL DRINKER

Anyone drinking over fourteen units a week is, by definition, drinking harmfully. So even if you are comforted by the notion that you never drink enough to become drunk, just less than a bottle and a half of wine over the course of the week should be considered the limit. For many people, however, drinking is not something they engage in for the taste; rather it is for the effect and the relief of emotional flat lining. For these people, one or two small glasses of wine on any given occasion would not fulfil their desire to temporarily alter their state of mind and therefore the government guidelines soon fall by the wayside. In this current climate where wine is consumed on a daily basis for many, it is certainly not unusual to fall into this category of 'harmful drinker.'

HAZARDOUS DRINKER

This is the stage before extreme alcohol dependency, where at least one bottle of wine a night is consumed. The recommended weekly number of units for women is fourteen, and yet with one bottle of wine amounting to approximately ten, a situation can easily be reached where between seventy and one hundred units becomes the weekly standard. If everyone else in your social group appears to be consuming in large volume too, it can feel as though this level of exceptionally heavy drinking is entirely normal.

Most people never measure in units, only by the glass, and the standard pub glass size has increased in recent years to 250ml. Three glasses at this volume equates to a bottle, and three glasses per day also increases the risk of breast cancer by approximately 50%.

Hazardous drinking is most often undertaken in the evenings, when the persuasive reasoning of 'I deserve it' becomes a daily mantra, and every night then dissolves into autopilot mode, the mind growing increasingly foggy and fuzzy. God forbid the hazardous drinker should ever need to drive to an emergency, or even have an early start in the car; one bottle of wine takes eleven hours to leave the system, which doesn't bode well for the school run.

Alcohol dependency is progressive; at this stage the slide down the slippery slope is well underway. Blackouts are beginning to kick in, and women who drink heavily can also experience a rise in testosterone levels of up to 60% – this aggression often plays a big part in the downward spiral; it's out of character, it doesn't fit with the fantasy women often cling to that wine-drinking equals sophistication and glamour, and it can lead to bouts of verbal and/or physical aggression.

MAINTENANCE DRINKER

This is another form of very hazardous drinking defined by a constant, and often secret, style of alcohol consumption. Never totally sober but always topped up, these women often appear to drink little when out socially. Many pre-load before leaving the house and become adept at managing their moods and outward signs of intoxication, as the thought of being ousted as an 'alkie' is, to the maintenance drinker, abhorrent. The degree of control displayed during any social event can be rather impressive, although as soon as things have been taken care of and it's home time again, the secret bottle is sought out from its hiding place and alcohol levels are topped up once more, the drinker alone and numb.

In the case of Sarah's business, this type of drinker often only resorts to asking for help as a result of being breathalysed or because another unforeseen but catastrophic event directly related to their alcohol intake has occurred. Openness frequently does not come easily to the maintenance drinker and thus for many, it can be difficult to even acknowledge that a problem exists.

HEAVILY-DEPENDENT DRINKER

By this stage, drinking spirits at breakfast-time no longer seems shocking and is perceived as a necessary pick-me-up to put an end to the shakes as well as to enable the drinker to attempt to proceed with even the smallest of everyday tasks. Once the hit of the alcohol has reached the spot, the daily drinking tango begins again. Defensive, broken, and lost, life cannot be maintained for long once this point has been reached, and it is

185

only a matter of time before either an alcohol-related accident or illness ensures this type of drinker pays the ultimate price for such excessive consumption.

Although there are more subtle elements to these categories, we hope that in describing the above various 'types' of drinker, you, the reader, will be able to recognise your own drinking patterns and hopefully begin working on a plan of action to combat the reasons why you have developed your own particular alcohol dependency.

THE METAPHORICAL CLIFF

Many women demonstrate a pattern of behaviour which stems from their transitional years of growing from a teenager to an adult. During that young and vulnerable phase of life, girls are bombarded by imagery of super slim, super beautiful, and sexually provocative females, glaring out at them from all directions – the cinema screen, television, magazines, and the world of pop music – leaving them in no doubt that there is just one ideal of feminine perfection in Western society and if they fall short of it, they are falling short in life.

Feelings of inadequacy frequently lead to self-abuse which many women secretly slip into the habit of during their teens and twenties (self-harming, eating disorders, alcohol and/or drug abuse) in an effort to fit in and feel more in control. In doing so, a cycle of self-victimisation often forms, resulting in an increased sense of fragility and defencelessness, not to mention the damage caused to physical health which only serves to make us feel even weaker and less able.

Fast forward a few years when the reality of long-term relationships, a frequently uneven division of domestic labour, the juggling of children and work commitments and a now less-than-great body image as a result of pregnancy and childbirth, can push many women to enter into deep levels of depression and anxiety. Add to this list the hormonal upheavals we endure at various stages of adulthood and life commonly begins to seem like one massive uphill struggle, and with a multitude of chores and hassles to overcome each day there can appear to be little in the way of light relief.

Further along the trajectory of family life are the often forgotten and almost invisible women whose children have grown up and flown the nest. For years these women have always loved their family and enjoyed being Mum, but have nonetheless looked forward to the freedom of being child-free once again, daydreaming of travelling and indulging in spontaneity with masses of 'me time.'

For these women, alcohol may have never been much of an issue prior to the children deserting the nest, but the sudden and cavernous void which demands to be filled can push a light or moderate alcohol usage into more of a dependency. The long term dream has finally arrived but after decades of concentrating on everyone else's happiness, women in this position commonly find it impossible to grant themselves all that they have longed for on so many occasions. The liberation swiftly disappears and the feelings of redundancy set in.

And for all of the above women, the wine crutch often appears to provide a much longed-for respite from deep emotional pain.

Piling the regrets and self-loathing associated with regular, heavy drinking on top of the already-present feelings of low self-worth which so many women are weighted down by, and the outcome is not surprising; someone who is deeply unhappy and who has no concept of what life is truly supposed to be like, only the notion that each day is a struggle and the one tiny element of joy in it is to be found in the booze aisle of the local supermarket. However, because alcohol is a depressant ('yeah, yeah, heard that one before, but what about the fact that I feel so happy with such a sense of release whenever I have that first glass?' I hear you cry) it actually contributes to any underlying depression. It could even be the root cause of a person's depression.

The heavy burden of any personal sorrows which are festering in the mind, together with the desperately low self-esteem which often begins all those years ago as a teenager, become buried deeper as each night of drinking passes by in a blur. Our problems are not resolved by drinking alcohol; through excessive alcohol consumption we fail to address them satisfactorily and these unresolved issues frequently then affect our everyday moods and how we interact with those around us.

We live in a culture in which alcohol is so pervasive, where every large-scale event from sporting tournaments to music festivals is saturated with booze. So overtly present and acceptable, it can seem almost unimaginable to exclude this, the most socially acceptable of all drugs, from your life for good. But many people are doing just that, and it seems that around the time we reach our thirties and forties is a common trigger point for assessing exactly who we are and what we want from life, including whether our ever-increasing reliance on alcohol is particularly conducive to a happy and fulfilling existence.

There is a common theme to be found in the way many women regard themselves in our society, characterised by strong feelings of not being good enough. But exactly why do we so regularly put ourselves down in this way when we are

188

simultaneously bringing up the next generation, pursuing a career, running a household and supporting our friends, partners and other family members in a number of different ways?

Why do we not, in reality, give ourselves a huge collective pat on the back for our incredible multi-tasking skills, our strength of character and our ability to achieve so much? We should be bursting with pride at all the things we accomplish each and every day but instead, more often than not, we tear ourselves apart with criticism and hit the wine in some misguided effort to alleviate the emotional upset we are experiencing inside.

The outstanding and remarkable are regularly underplayed, while the unimportant and insignificant are often blown out of all proportion forming the basis of long-standing and overly-critical perceptions of who we are. And out comes the wine; the self-medicating, tinkling sound of liquid poured into our favourite wine glass soothing us into believing that we are ameliorating our stressful worlds, when in actuality we are adding to our problems – in a big way.

Take the two of us as a microcosm of the common phenomenon of women failing to fulfil their potential, so caught up as many of us are in concentrating on our perceived failures as opposed to celebrating our successes; we both spent decades of our lives underachieving as a direct result of drinking. Since cutting out alcohol, life has become a series of positive confirmations of the best aspects of our characters. Whether this is manifested in more rewarding relationships with family and friends, increased productivity and success in the workplace, or by the easier attainment of personal goals, we cannot stress enough how living alcohol-free has really helped us to beat long-standing feelings of low self-worth and given us back a whole host of reasons to finally like ourselves.

Imagine if women all over the world took this bold step of ditching alcohol and were able to develop their inner selves fully, minus the constrictive and self-esteem destroying influences of ethanol; we could witness a sober revolution. When feminism began to fully gather pace in the 1970s, did anyone ever imagine that the wine manufacturers would embark on a mission to market their produce at Western women in such an effective way that by the late 1990s we would be actively sowing the seeds of our own unhappiness though the sheer volume of the stuff we were guzzling en masse? Alcohol abuse robs those who engage in it of their sense of self, their compassion for other people and of the energy and drive to chase their dreams and aspirations.

Take Pam who stopped drinking a year ago, and subsequently joined a cycling club which hits the Peak District in Derbyshire on a regular basis throughout the summer months for long bike rides (and I mean long – 100 km!). Her level of fitness has never been greater, and her self-esteem has been provided with a huge injection of oomph as she cannot believe quite what she has achieved every time she completes one of these massive group rides, keeping pace with scores of others clad in Lycra as she aims to smash her personal best, month on month.

Or Sue, a woman in her fifties who was facing redundancy and spent several months really hitting the bottle in a misguided effort to numb the problem away before deciding to accept the severance pay, quit drinking and set up her own consultancy business.

With masses of new-found energy and her depression now completely eradicated, Sue's little empire is going from strength to strength, and her self-worth has gone through the roof as a result. Since quitting alcohol, Sue has also ridden a zip wire across the River Tyne, and danced, sober of course, in high heels until the early hours at her daughter's wedding.

And Mikki, who, in a past life drank a bottle of wine a night in order to try and cope with the stress she suffered in her old teaching job, quit drinking altogether, handed in her notice and established a business with her husband. Now back in control of her life following the decision to lose her emotional crutch on alcohol, Mikki loves every minute she spends working on her burgeoning empire, has relocated for business purposes, and the stress and anxiety are well on their way to disappearing completely too. Her new hobby of crocheting helps her unwind in the evenings and the number of items she has created is growing at the same rate as her feelings of self-worth.

What these women have collectively done is to step off a metaphorical cliff edge into an unknown vacuum of living without alcohol, and found themselves free-falling directly into the person they were meant to be all along, the one who was hiding beneath all their erstwhile excessive drinking. The simple truth is that we cannot ever know just how strong, how ambitious, or how compassionate we really are while we are filling up on rocket fuel each night. And despite a sadly not unusual tendency to sabotage both mind and body through over-eating, under-eating, drinking excessively, self-harming, or doing drugs, when reality is allowed to take over, women usually discover that life minus the old crutches is a million times more enjoyable than their old existence and not the dreaded, scary world that they imagined it would be during darker days. Letting go of the alcohol crutch means empowering yourself.

ESSENTIALITY

A major fear about becoming alcohol-free is that without booze the ability to have fun and let one's hair down may be lost, and that it has only been the alcohol all along which has enabled these characteristics to come to the fore, rather than any essential qualities that lie naturally within us. In the interim period between the last drink and being completely comfortable as a non-drinker, many people linger in something of a No Man's Land in terms of how to act in social situations, as they are no longer drinking and thus adopting the false persona that booze brings out in people, but neither do they really know who they are without alcohol. Discovering yourself after years of habitual and heavy drinking takes a while, there's no getting around that fact.

However, a big mistake when approaching a new alcohol-free life is to put the brakes on in any way with regards to your essentiality – letting go of the wine crutch does not mean that you should no longer enjoy yourself, listen to loud music whenever the fancy takes you, dance at parties, hold your own in a heated debate at a dinner party, or laugh until the tears roll down your face at a joke someone tells you.

Feeling free enough to act in a carefree manner and able to lose your inhibitions without drinking excessive amounts of alcohol can take a little practice but when it happens, the joy derived from finally allowing yourself to be YOU without any of the falsity or the negative implications of heavy alcohol consumption, is monumental.

We, as human beings, were not designed half-finished, unable to be truly happy or to have fun unless we were topped up with booze. As children we were mostly carefree with the ability to leap into a fun-filled situation at a moment's notice; believing that we need alcohol in order to enjoy life is nonsensical and anyone who has successfully and happily ditched the booze would support the notion that a person's essentiality only truly comes alive once the wine has been left behind.

A HELPING HAND

Ultimately, living alcohol-free should never be about willpower, gritting your teeth and using any desperate trick in the book to get you through the day without hitting the wine cellar, BUT in the early days of sobriety both your mind and body are adjusting to life without an addictive substance and therefore you will experience cravings. Below are some ideas from members of the Soberistas community on how to survive those initial few days and/or weeks minus the Wine Witch:

"The most important tip for me is remembering that any physical craving for booze only lasts for ten minutes – no idea why it's exactly that, but to distract for ten minutes is not too painful. In the early days I used an egg timer to focus my mind ..."

"Keep a little tube of toothpaste and brush in your handbag – brushing my teeth took the desire for wine away, and it was especially handy for when I finished work; that seemed to be a major trigger for me."

"My tip to those starting out would be to try to delay that first drink – by five minutes if necessary (for me committing to a

whole day was overwhelming to start with, but minutes I could do), then delay it again by another five minutes and again and again – bite-size chunks in which you choose not to drink. Before you know it, those little chunks have added up to the whole evening, it's bedtime and you're AF."

"Envisage trying to achieve a life of sobriety like running in a hurdles race. If you concentrate on the second or third hurdle you'll fall over the first! One at a time and you'll get to the end successfully!"

"I buy expensive chocolates, cordials, coconut water, and an array of beautiful magazines to fill the treat-shaped hole. Oh and I drink from elegant glasses."

"Not drinking needs to be The Number 1 Priority."

"My tip is the only thing that has really worked for me and I am 10 weeks alcohol-free today! The constant support of others on Soberistas made me realise I was not alone on this journey which at the beginning was a fearful one as I truly believed I would never be able to get rid of this poisonous habit. It was hearing from others who had made the journey and achieved becoming AF and hearing from some who had slipped but picked themselves up and carried on. Not being the only one made a huge difference for me."

"The thing that helps me is to always remember the phrase, 'Play the movie to the end.' The idea of a glass of cold wine on a warm summer's evening is sometimes tempting but if I fast-forward in my head to 11pm, I see the definite and depressing

outcome; me hammered, staggering about, probably about to throw up, and arguing with my husband. It just isn't worth taking the risk of that first glass."

"For me, the uppermost thought in my mind for every day is acceptance – accepting that I have the problem first of all, but also accepting the fact that we can't change anything else but ourselves and our own behaviour. Along the way we come across so many obstacles and difficult people and situations that we can do absolutely nothing about ... it's life, it happens. We have to accept it for what it is and do the best possible job we can do for ourselves."

"Someone told me to start a 'count your blessings jar' – you put the money in the jar that you would have spent on drinking. Then you buy yourself something nice. It works for me. My jar is clear glass so I can see the growing pile of money in there every morning."

"My advice would be to really take it slowly and give yourself 'you time.' In life we don't concentrate and spend enough time on us which results in us getting stressed. Taking some time every day to live in the moment really helps me, whether it is going for a run, doing crochet, or just sitting with my glass of tonic! It is when I don't do this that I end up with the occasional wobble!!! So 'me time' is my number one tip."

"Eat earlier. If you can't eat at teatime, then snack – that puts the craving off too. Or just eat little and often, but the key is to never allow yourself to feel hungry."

"The best tip from me has to be joining Soberistas, especially as it's available 24/7. Being able to remain anonymous has allowed me to be completely honest for the first time about my relationship with alcohol, and that has been so liberating for me. I love the solidarity, friendship, support, shared experiences, encouragement, and understanding which was so unexpected. I feel quite determined not to blip as it would feel to me like wasting all the support from everyone here who has so helped me be strong."

THE BIG REVEAL

As discussed in earlier chapters of the book, informing friends and family of a decision to become a non-drinker can be the cause of worry for many who are new to sobriety. Alcohol is a hugely socially acceptable drug and for the vast percentage of the Western population, every holiday, celebration, night out, barbeque, party, or quiet evening in spent watching a DVD, would not be complete without a few alcoholic drinks to imbibe.

As a result, 'coming out' as a non-drinker may be worthy of a little consideration before you reveal your new commitment to alcohol-free living to anyone who will listen. Some people make the decision to slightly bend the truth about the fact that they have ditched the booze, employing such reasons as weight loss or they are adopting a generally healthier lifestyle which includes becoming a non-drinker. Others choose to keep schtum, opting for non-alcoholic drinks when they are out socially without making a big deal of it – many non-drinkers discover that the people whose company they're in fail to notice after a certain time has passed, such is the effect of their own alcohol consumption in that it makes people less observant.

Being the designated driver is always an easy option, although you may not wish to rely on this as an explanation long-term; similarly, a course of antibiotics is an age-old excuse for refusing an alcoholic drink but it is not a reason which can be used for ever.

The final decision regarding letting your friends and family know that you no longer drink alcohol is yours to make and nobody else can know what will work best for you, in your own specific set of circumstances. We strongly feel, however, that although excuses and little white lies will buy you a limited amount of time, which may be helpful in the initial few weeks as you come to terms with all the changes this new lifestyle will bring, the best option for many reasons is to be truthful.

There is in certain people's minds a stigma attached to being a non-drinker – the most obvious explanation for this is that by your not drinking, their own alcohol consumption is highlighted, and perhaps unwantedly so. But by employing excuses as to why you no longer drink, you are perpetrating the idea that those who are teetotal are unusual and strange. If many more people take the healthy and positive step to eradicate booze from their lives, and crucially they are not afraid to tell people exactly that, then steps are being taken towards de-stigmatizing non-drinkers and normalising living without the alcohol crutch, just as regular binge-drinking is currently perceived to be acceptable currently.

You could try using one of the following explanations, successfully road-tested by ourselves and our clients:

"I don't drink because I felt that I lacked the ability to recognise when I'd had enough."

"I stopped drinking because I wanted to be a better parent – alcohol made me snappy and irritable and I didn't think that was fair on my kids."

"I always seemed to end up drinking way more than the government guidelines, and I got scared about the health implications."

"Whenever I drank, I got inordinately pissed and embarrassed myself – I got bored with looking stupid and waking up full of regret."

"I gave up alcohol for a few weeks just to take a break from it but I enjoyed the effects that being teetotal had on me so much that I just never got round to starting again."

"Call me vain but I started to notice how puffy my face had become and how much weight I was putting on, both of which I knew were as a result of drinking too much wine. I wanted to try and look younger and fresher-faced and so I quit."

By utilising one of the above reasons for becoming alcohol-free, you can ensure that you are getting the truth out there (which is important, not only because it makes life easier for you in the long run, but it also promotes being a non-drinker as the positive lifestyle choice it is, rather than a terrible burden of shame which some have been unfortunate to be made to feel they carry as a result of stopping drinking), freeing you up to get along with the joy and liberation to be found in the act of rejecting the Wine Witch on a permanent basis.

Ultimately, embarking upon a booze-free lifestyle is a decision that can only be made by you. Choosing to live alcohol-free can present its challenges in the initial period of adjustment, but it is our belief that as a long-term solution to a multitude of problems that so many women encounter with regards to low self-esteem, lack of confidence, anxiety and depression, ditching the Wine Witch makes an awful lot of sense.

By adopting a life that doesn't feature alcohol, we are empowering ourselves with freedom of choice, nurturing a calmer mental state which helps us to be more patient as parents and more understanding as partners and friends. In stepping out of the alcohol trap, we can liberate ourselves from its many destructive effects that have prevented us from fulfilling our potential ever since we began to drink heavily, and can focus our energies on making the most out of life, and who we really are.

Becoming a non-drinker means climbing back
into the driving seat of your life, and enables YOU
to become a part of THE SOBER REVOLUTION.

Disclaimer

For many people, there is no substitute for professional therapy
with a counsellor who specialises in alcohol addiction. This
book is not a replacement for this, or any other type of
recognised alcohol addiction support/therapy, but an additional
support resource that may complement your other endeavours
to control your consumption of alcohol. If you are struggling
with an alcohol dependency or are at all worried about your
alcohol consumption, please discuss with your GP in the first
instance.

For contact details of alcohol support groups, please visit the
Soberistas website.

Your Six Week Plan

Join The Sober Revolution –
and call time on wine o'clock

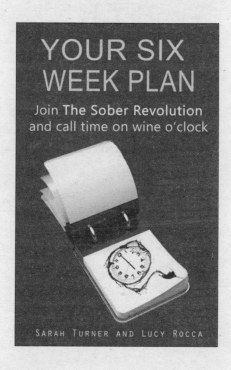

Packed with great tips, inspirational quotes, delicious alcohol-free drinks recipes, and expert advice on how to beat cravings, you can use the book like a diary, creating a personal record of your own journey to alcohol-free living.

For other **Accent Press** titles
please visit

www.accentpress.co.uk